CHAPTER I.

INTRODUCTION.

Although it is evident to my mind that the world is growing more healthy and more moral with every generation—speaking of civilized nations—it is still, as all agree, in a most pitiful state as regards both moral and physical health. The two are indissolubly associated, notwithstanding the glaring exceptions which are, indeed, more apparent than real, and it is difficult to appreciate which leads—whether man grows more healthy as his moral tone improves or more moral as his physical state is exalted. Both are, in fact, constantly acting and reacting upon each other. Few people withdraw themselves from the influence of disease-producing habits, who do not first come to hate disease as a symptom of disobedience to the laws governing their organism. The pain of an aching head is not sufficient, generally, although it may discount the tortures of the damned, to determine the sufferer to live a better life; but when he comes to know the fact that the disorder is needless, brought upon himself by violation of law, and that it is the normal office of pain to warn of danger; then, if he be conscientious, instead of cursing his suffering, he will feel ashamed of his sin, and endeavor to learn the laws of life and obey them.

"In days gone by and not far away, there was a very general impression with the people that sickness and the death which so often follows it were of divine origination and ordainment. No person who might be sick blamed himself for it; certainly no one was held by the community of which he was a member, as in any sense responsible or blameworthy because of his death by sickness. It was believed that for reasons thoroughly justifiable, but incomprehensible to the mind of man, the Supreme Ruler saw fit to manifest His modes and methods of government, either providential or punitive, by taking away the health or the life of those who became sick, or who being sick died of their sickness.

"This notion, though not so prevalent as formerly, still lingers in the popular mind and lies hidden away in the select circles of religious people, occasionally to be brought forth and urged upon public consideration with emphasis, when some person is taken sick and remains for many months and perhaps years an invalid, or when one taken sick suddenly dies.

"There is no basis in science nor in religion for this impression. It never rose, it never can rise, to the dignity or worthiness of an idea; it must always dwell, no matter who entertains it, on the low level of irrational impression. Its basis is error, not knowledge; its superstructure is superstition. By and by, when mankind shall reach such a degree of rational development as to understand that human life has its laws, and that human health is but the legitimate outcome of the operation of these laws, and that every human being of every tribe and kindred and tongue, is born to live on earth under such minute and careful providential arrangements as to hold within him, at his starting, great securities and guarantees of the very highest order, for the continuance of his life up to a definite period, and that by reason of this inherent capability, he is entitled to live to the full measure of his endowment, this foolish, I may say wicked, notion, that God kills people will disappear. When it shall be abandoned, the sickness which now is so common everywhere, and the deaths which now so frequently result, will cease, and human beings will live from birth to death by old age, casualties, and accidents one side, as surely as the seasons come and go."[1]

[1] "The Absurdity of Sickness," by James C. Jackson, M.D.

Few people have any just conception of the prevalence of disease even in their own midst—among their own kindred; and this is simply because it never absurdly happens that all those who are subject to illnesses are "attacked" at the same time. When any large proportion are down at once, the doctors call it an *epidemic*, and it is attributed to a "wave"—an epizootic or influenza wave, for example, according as the victims are horses or men (the poor animals depend upon the elevated race for their habits, and never have disease except these are unphysiological),—when, in fact, the so-called epidemic, whether it be scarlet or yellow fever, diphtheria, or what not, is the result chiefly of the uniformly bad living habits of our people and their consequent predisposition to sickness. I do not ignore the influence of contagion in certain disorders, but assert that no person in *prime physical condition* is ever made sick by transient contact with the so-called contagious diseases.

"There can be no doubt," says Dr. Moore, "of the inherent effort of the system to preserve its integrity and to resist and overcome the effects of morbid influences. And when the system is properly organized and perfect in its physiological functions, it has the power to accomplish this (unless these obnoxious influences are so overwhelming as to destroy life at once) in a prompt and complete manner, unaided by any external influences whatsoever, so that health will be maintained and all injurious action of disease-producing causes unconsciously and successfully averted. But if instead of such a properly organized and healthy system, we have formed an incomplete and inferior grade of structural organization, and consequently an enervated nervous system, resulting from imperfect and deficient nutrition, such as evidently exists in the scorbutic diathesis (the effect of deficiency in vegetable food), or as must result from habitual or frequent digestive disturbances, this endeavor to resist or avert disease, will be necessarily so enfeebled that it will be impossible for the system, by its own inherent and unaided energy, either to ward off or to overcome the effects of disease-producing agents. This protective and restorative effort, if not sustained by a high character of structural organization and active nervous energy, must be followed, therefore, as a natural consequence, by an exhaustion of vital power; in which condition there would be evidently an increased susceptibility to all morbific influences, and a marked predisposition to any exciting causes of disease which might be brought to bear upon it.

"It is well known that certain individuals are more severely affected by any ascertained cause of disease than others; and also that the same exciting cause may at one time produce serious disturbance of health, while at another, and under precisely the same conditions, as far as known, no injurious effect is produced. How frequently do we observe during the same epidemic, as, for instance, scarlet fever, measles, diphtheria (and even of sporadic forms of disease), a marked difference in the character and severity of individual cases. Even in members of the same family, under apparently similar conditions, some are stricken down with the most malignant form of one of these diseases, while others may, at the same time, be but slightly affected by it, or perhaps entirely escape an attack. It can not be that they who are the most severely affected receive a larger or a stronger dose of the morbific agent which has produced the disorder, than the others, and that the disease-producing influence, in consequence of larger quantity or greater strength and power, acts with more severity and force on one than on another. For, leaving out of consideration all effects of existing predisposition, we know that a person unprotected by a previous attack or by vaccination, would be, in all probability, just as severely affected by the contagious influence of a case of small-pox, whether he was exposed for a few moments or for several hours; and besides, it would make no difference whether the case happened to be a mild one or of a more malignant form.

"It is, therefore, difficult to account for this variable operation of disease-producing agents, unless we admit the existence of such a latent predisposition as that already mentioned, and acknowledge that the system, at the time of exposure to disease-producing causes, is thereby made more or less susceptible to their effects in proportion to the development of such a predisposition. The less the power of resistance and the greater the degree of impressibility, the more aggravated will be the character of every disease which affect the system while it is thus predisposed; or, in other words, the severity of the disease will be proportionate to the degree of departure from the standard of health."[2]

[2] "Predisposition and Typhoid Tendency," by Thomas Moore, M.D. Philadelphia.

Predisposition is that state of susceptibility produced by the continued operation of the predisposing cause. *Exciting causes* are those which tend to the immediate development of diseases, especially in a system already having a predisposition thereto.

But in my opening remarks, I had in view, particularly, the common sicknesses that prevail among us, and which are not classed as contagious. Not one in the thousand of our population *so lives* as to feel an assurance of absolute health for, say, a single month, much less for the coming twelve months. There are, however, among the class I shall hold up as examples to my readers, further on, individuals who would be willing to stake their lives on their ability to meet any engagement depending upon a mental and physical state, equal to that enjoyed at the present moment, on any day, week, or month, during the next year or ten years; and every ordinarily healthy person, who can fairly be called a free agent, ought to be able to feel such an assurance in his own case; and if he be at middle-age, or under, and afflicted with ailments, other than organic and incurable, he should be able to count with certainty on being a better man, physically as well as morally, ten years hence than he is to-day.

But how is it in practice? Why, even our national salutation (which is, also, about the same among all civilized nations) is significant in this connection, as we shall observe, further on: if sickness was the exception and not the rule, health would not be the stock question everywhere and always—the principal theme of conversation—as it is now. People seem to delight in a subject that they know nothing about, like a good old Methodist preacher I once knew, who said on one occasion, at prayer-meeting: "I love to talk about religion—I have so little of it."

We talk about enjoying good health, and some of my readers would, I dare say, make the claim for themselves, although too well aware of occasional lapses, and indeed the great proportion of our people, in spite of heredity, might obtain, and rest secure in, a high state of health; but, living as they do, a truly sound person is almost the rarest thing in the world.

"How are you?" is the question on meeting an acquaintance. "First-rate, although I have my old sick headaches occasionally." Another replies, "Pretty well, *now*—have just had a touch of neuralgia—you know I always had that now and then." Another has a "bad cold in the head." Smith enjoys good health, although "troubled a good deal with dyspepsia, constipation, etc.," which means that he is constantly annoyed by symptoms inseparable from his disease. Jones is "tip-top," with an occasional "attack" of cholera-morbus, or a bilious spell. Brown "never was better in his life," but could tell you of a fearful sickness last spring—"like to have died," and no wonder—he had three drug doctors and a gallstone! Robinson is "tough as a knot"—just now—since getting cleaned out by erysipelas—an eruption of the accumulated poison resulting from his bad habits. It was a fearful "attack," as he says! "The doctor called it the worst case he ever saw—my head was swelled so I couldn't see for weeks—used up a bushel of cranberries in poultices, when I had counted on having cranberry sauce all winter—did not get a spoonful." Of course Robinson exaggerates about the quantity of cranberries.

Tom, one of the healthiest-looking specimens, recently had typhoid fever and came near dying. Mrs. Dick had "slow fever" the past summer and managed to keep it a-going for three months. She says it was a dreadful "attack"; and she tries to explain it by saying that several years ago, she had it every summer for three summers, and "it generally leaves the seeds in the system!" Harry's wife had stoppage and inflammation of the bowels—a deadly sickness for six months, entailing infinite distress on the large family that needed her about so much. "The doctor's big bill isn't paid yet," she mourns, "and mercy only knows when it will be." She has always been a well woman, so-called, has always seemed pretty well until this terrible disease "attacked" her.

The list is endless, of the so-called healthy ones who have been from time to time "attacked" with one disorder or another and recovered,—while the mortality reports from week to week tell the final story of the premature taking off of thousands of men, women, and children who, although always regarded by themselves and friends as healthy, have suffered the death-penalty after a longer or shorter imprisonment.

How often we hear such remarks as this: "I never was so surprised in my life as I was to hear of Miss Blank's death—perfect picture of health—fat, hearty, red-cheeked—the last person in the world I would have thought of dying." This shows how much the people know about health. Ninety-nine in a hundred would have called this young lady a specimen of health, when, in fact, any expert would have known that she was a typhoid subject—almost sure to be down with it sooner or later, and, with her whole physical conditions so against her, that recovery would be almost a miracle, *under the prevailing system of treatment.* Just recall the scores of cases where you, my dear reader, have been surprised at the death of this or that friend, "always so strong and well." In fact, this is so common that we expect to be surprised continually, and are not much surprised when we are!

How many healthy-born infants die before their first year is reached—babies that for months are mistakenly regarded as pictures of health—"never knew a sick day until they were attacked" with cholera-infantum, scarlatina, or something else. They are crammed with food, made gross with fat, and for a time are active and cunning, the delight of parents and friends—and then, after a season of constipation, a season of chronic vomiting, and a season of cholera-infantum, the little emaciated skeletons are buried in the ground away from the sight of those who have literally *loved them to death.* This is the fate of one-third of all the children born. As a rule, babies are fed as an ignorant servant feeds the cook-stove—filling the fire-box so full, often, that the covers are raised, the stove smokes and gases at every hole, and the fire is either put out altogether, or, if there is combustion of the whole body of coals, the stove is rapidly burned out and destroyed. With baby, "overheating" means the fever that consumes him, and, in "putting out the fire," too often the fire of life goes out also.[3]

[3] For a thorough discussion of this question see the author's work on Infant Dietetics, entitled "How to Feed the Baby" New York: Fowler & Wells.

"For the preservation of life God has ordained certain laws to be observed, the neglect of which necessarily brings disease and premature death." Hence it is that if any of us are sick—except from accidents or congenital causes—it is our own fault. If we have dyspepsia, and the endless afflictions resulting from this parent of diseases, it is our own fault —either of ignorance or carelessness. If neuralgia, "sciatica," rheumatism, gout, or sick-headache afflicts us, we can thank ourselves; for the simple question is—whether it will "pay" to keep clear of them? It is all very fine to bowl along without thought; to eat, drink, and breathe, without using our brains or consciences, and to shun the best products of the brains of others who make this subject the study of their lives, and when the inevitable sickness comes shift the responsibility on to the Lord. It is rank blasphemy, nevertheless.

In the struggle of life, when so many of His children are engrossed in the vital question of bread-winning; when to obtain the mere necessities of life, or, at most, these and the ordinary comforts, requires all the time, early and late, of so large a portion of the human family, it is not to be supposed that the Creator designed that the due and proper care of the body—its development and the maintenance of a healthy state—should be a matter of such complications as to be beyond the comprehension of ordinary mortals, or require the expenditure of an amount of time that would prove embarrassing to all, and totally impossible to many. Nor should Christians conclude that an "all-wise, all-merciful, and all-powerful Father" designed that the creatures formed in "His own likeness" should alone, of all created beings, be necessarily subject to the multifarious forms of disease, that in fact, under present conditions, do so continually afflict them. Happily such conclusions are not borne out by rational experience; for, in practice, it is found that not only is less trouble and expense required to keep well, than to pursue a course that is promotive of disease; and to get well when disease is really fastened upon us, than to continue the general regimen that has worked the mischief, and seek to counteract it by poisonous drugs; but in fact it has been clearly shown by innumerable living examples, that neither much time, trouble, or expense is necessary to maintain the body in a state of absolute health—perfect ease and comfort—when once this state has been reached, or to restore to comparative health a large proportion of "miserable sinners" who, without a radical change in their mode of life, must continue to suffer from their self-inflicted pains.

It requires no more time to breathe pure than impure air—and no more time or expense to obtain it: it is as free as air, and will fill our homes, without money and without price, unless we seal them against its admission. The poorest factory-operative that goes by the bell, can with a pint of water and a single towel, if need be, take a three-minute bath any or every morning, if he appreciates its importance and is conscientious in his living. It costs no more to eat enough than to over-indulge the appetite, as is the universal rule, high and low, until nausea and lack of appetite compel abstinence or moderation. It costs money to poison the system with beer or tobacco, and thus shorten one's life and impair its usefulness, and transmit evil moral and physical tendencies to his offspring, but it is a ten-fold saving to keep clear of these evils. And so it proves throughout the list: it is cheap to keep well, and dear to get sick.

"So to observe Nature as to learn her laws and obey them, is to observe the commandments of the Lord to do them. It has so long been the habit to exalt the mind as the noble, spiritual, and immortal part, at the expense of the body, as the vile, material and mortal part, that, while it is not thought at all strange that every possible care and attention should be given to mental cultivation, a person who should give the same sort of careful attention to his body would be thought somewhat meanly of. And yet I am sure that a wise man who would ease best the burden of life, can not do better than watchfully to keep undefiled and holy—that is, healthy—the noble temple of his body. Is it not a glaring inconsistency that men should pretend to fall into ecstasies of admiration of the temples which they have built with their own hands, and to claim reverence for their ruins, and, at the same time, should have no reverence for, or should actually speak contemptuously of, that most complex, ingenious, and admirable structure which the human body is? However, if they really neglect it, it is secure of its revenge—no one will come to much by his most strenuous mental exercises, except upon the basis of a good organization; for a sound body is assuredly the foundation of a sound mind." (Maudsley).

That there is need of a radical change in the study and practice of medicine, is well known among those who have examined the subject with any degree of thoroughness. A prominent defect is thus described by the eminent Dr. Combe: "The little regard," he says, "which has hitherto been paid to the laws of the human constitution, as the true basis on which our attempts to improve the condition of man ought to rest, will be obvious from the fact, that, notwithstanding the direct uses, to which a knowledge of the conditions, which regulate the healthy action of the bodily organs, may be applied in the prevention, detection, and treatment of disease, there is scarcely a medical school in this country (Great Britain)[4] in which any special provision is made for teaching it.... The prominent aim of medicine being to discriminate, and to cure *diseases*, both the teacher and the student naturally fix upon that as their chief object, and are consequently apt to overlook the indirect (!) but substantial aid, which an acquaintance with the laws of health is calculated to afford, in restoring the sick as well as in preserving the healthy from disease." The use of the word "indirect," in this connection shows how far Dr. Combe, himself, was from having a true comprehension of the importance of hygienic knowledge. Although individuals, here and there, finally work out this knowledge for themselves, it is generally late in life, when long years of blundering practice have forced it upon them. Hear what some of the wise old heads say on this point:

[4] Some advance has been made in this direction of late, but the outlook is far from satisfactory; there is scarcely a college lecture-room but in deficient ventilation, or a lecturer whose living habits, and, consequently, personal health, do not cry aloud, "Physician, heal thyself."

A. H. Stevens, M.D.: "The older physicians grow, the more skeptical they become in the virtues of their own medicines." Prof. Willard Parker: "Of all sciences, medicine is the most unreliable." Prof E. H. Davis: "The vital effects of medicine are little understood." J. Mason Goode, M.D.: "The science of medicine is a barbarous jargon." Dr. Bostwick, author of "History of Medicine": "Every dose of medicine is a blind experiment." Prof. Evans, M.D.: "The medical practice of the present day is neither philosophy nor common sense." It was the well-known remark of Dr. James Gregory, who added as much reputation to the medical school of the University of Edinburgh, as any other individual—that, "ninety-nine in the hundred medical 'facts' are medical lies, and that all medical theories are stark, staring nonsense." Dr. McClintock: "Mercury has made more cripples than all wars combined," and he might have added that the abuse of soda or potassa in its present various forms is destroying myriads of stomachs every year beyond redemption. Sir Astley Cooper, the most famous physician and surgeon of the age: "The science of medicine is founded on conjecture and improved by murder." Oliver Wendell Holmes said before a medical class in 1861 "The disgrace of medicine has been that colossal system of self-deception, in obedience to which mines have been emptied of their cankering minerals, the vegetable kingdom robbed of all its growth, the entrails of animals taxed for their impurities, the poison bags of reptiles drained of their venom, and all the conceivable abominations thus obtained thrust down the throats of human beings, suffering from some fault of organization, nourishment, or vital stimulation."

That the practice of medicine to-day is not what it should be, is due largely to the position of the laity on this point—their aversion to taking advice instead of medicine. They will consider the question of prevention, in the shape of anti-bilious pills, for example, but not at the expense of their lawful follies. If indeed physicians, generally, knew enough about the natural laws to retain their own health, how could they all derive an income from teaching the simple method by which all their neighbors would remain well? A patient, for example, is suffering pain, and sends for the doctor, who comes, examines, and finally says, "I find nothing serious here—this pain in the head will soon leave you—just keep about if you can; if not, remain quiet. Coming in from the fresh air, I observe that your room is very close, sufficient of itself to give you the headache—change the air and keep it pure; eat nothing more to-day: you are 'ahead of your stomach,' withal; in fact, that is the chief trouble. Take a quick sponge bath on retiring, and you will find yourself all right in the morning—you need no medicine." Do you fancy he would get another call from her, or from her friends through her influence? Her *head aches*, and she is incensed at such heartless nonsense. She sends for another doctor, who will probably be sharp enough to treat her *disposition*, and endeavor to "control the symptoms" instead of teaching her to remove the disease by removing its cause; he gives her a "quieting medicine"—something to deaden her senses; she has several days' illness, he gets several fees—as he ought, to be sure—and the good-will of the family; and so he rises in the profession, while the other falls into the shade unless he drops his hygienic nonsense. Thus, we observe, a premium on shrewdness and a tax on sincerity.

"It is notorious that in proportion to people's ignorance of their own constitutions and the true causes of disease, is their credulous confidence in pills, potions, and quackish absurdities, and while this ignorance continues, there will, of course, be plenty of doctors who will pander to it. And not the least of the benefits likely to follow the better diffusion of physiological and sanitary information will be the protection of the community from the numberless impostures of charlatanism, and a better discrimination of the qualifications of competent physicians."[5]

[5] "Physiology and Hygiene," Huxley and Youmans.

I take it that all are agreed as to the desirability of good health, although it is often said of a certain class of chronic invalids, that if they were to be deprived of the pleasure of croning over and detailing their symptoms, life would have no charms for them. But this is a provision of nature to prevent the meanest life from becoming altogether an unmitigated burden: when a person becomes so disordered physically that he has nothing else to enjoy, a certain depraved condition of mind is induced which enables him to extract a little satisfaction from dwelling upon and recounting his miseries! In contrast to such cases how gloriously shines out the example of the old lady who, on being interviewed by the minister, thus related her experiences: her husband had been long dead, leaving her with eight children, whom, through her own labor, she reared and educated. One after another all had died after lingering illnesses—the last, a son, the only support of her old age, had been recently buried; and, to crown all, the remnant of the little property left by her husband, had just passed from her possession—the uninsured buildings by fire, and the land by the foreclosure of the mortgage. "But," concluded the dear old soul, while her brow lightened and her eye kindled with enthusiasm, "thank the Lord, I have two teeth left, and praise and bless His holy name, they are opposite each other!" I pause to note an important lesson—the influence upon health, of prevalent good nature, and the habit, which may be cultivated, of looking on the bright side of things. "People ask me," says Old Sojourner Truth, "how I came to live so long and keep my mind, and I tell them that it is 'because I think of the great things of God, not little things.' I don't fritter my mind away in caring for trifles."

It has been elsewhere noted—the propensity of people in general for preferring medicine to advice. If the world were convinced that the writer possessed an unfailing remedy—a "medicine" that would cure every physical ailment and prevent disease, it would be demanded faster than it could be manufactured, though every gin-mill in the land were transformed into a laboratory for its production. No price would be deemed exorbitant, and, though the mixture were black as ink, and more nauseating than the vilest drug in our vile Materia Medica, it would still be gulped down as a child demolishes bon-bons, if it never failed in its efficacy.

We have only to look over the newspaper advertising columns to find scores of articles claiming to accomplish this, at the very reasonable price of 50 cents to $1.00 per bottle, "large bottles cheapest," and very agreeable to the taste; and evidence abounds in the shape of letters purporting to have been written by such as have, although given up by the doctors, been withdrawn from the grave (regardless of the rights of the heirs and undertakers)—restored to the busy walks of life—"and no change of diet necessary." Thousands upon thousands of otherwise sensible people are gulled into the belief that a few bottles of somebody's pretended "discovery," advertised in a yellow-covered almanac, will cure whatever ails them. There is something so fascinating about such literature that I would almost as soon place a package of Paris-green within reach of a baby as to put, say, a medical almanac, and more particularly a cookery-book with fancy dishes and medical lies alternating, in the hands of the average adult. There isn't one in fifty proof against them. Let the most robust Congressman spend one half-hour reading one of these "messages", with the endless variety of symptoms therein given, and the hundreds of letters of the blest—fabricated in the proprietor's office, or, at best, written by his victims during a temporary suppression of the symptoms—and, comparing his own feelings with those described, the chances are that he would soon be pouring down the medicine—convinced that it hit his case exactly. Why is this possible? Why, indeed, do we have a drug-store on every other corner, with shelves packed with the infamous "regular" and irregular remedies, simple and compound? Simply because ninety-five in the hundred men, women, and children so treat themselves that they do have, from day to day, or week to week, various symptoms more or less severe, all indicative of derangement of the bodily functions. And because of this the medicine-makers know that he who is the keenest and boldest in prostituting the art of printing, will reap the richest harvest, by reason of the ignorance and disease-producing habits of the people.

I will conclude these introductory remarks with the beautiful and impressive language of Professor Maudsley, the eminent English physician, especially celebrated in connection with the treatment of mental disorders, and who, as shown by the paragraph already quoted, emphasizes in the strongest manner, not only the intimate connection between the mind and the body—their interdependence the one with the other—but, also, the moral obligation of the *man* to learn and obey the laws which tend to exalt both:

"Notably the best rules for the conduct of life are the fruits of the best observations of men and things; the achievements of science are no more than the organized gains—orderly and methodically arranged—of an exact and systematic observation of the various departments of Nature; the noblest products of the arts are Nature ennobled through human means, the art itself being Nature. There are not two worlds—a world of Nature and a world of human nature—standing over against one another, in a sort of antagonism, but one world of Nature, in the orderly evolution of which human nature has its subordinate part. Disease, hallucinations, idiosyncrasies of whatever sort, are the product of disobedience to law—discordant notes in the Divine harmony, which result from an unskillful or careless touch. It should, then, be every man's steadfast aim, as a part of Nature, his patient work, to cultivate such entire sincerity of relations with it, so to think, feel, and act, always in intimate unison with it, that when the summons comes to surrender his mortal part to absorption into it, he does so, not fearfully, as to an enemy who has vanquished him, but trustfully, as to a mother who, when the day's task is done, bids him lie down to sleep."

CHAPTER II.

CONSUMPTION.

Among the causes of consumption it is usually held that inherited tendency is one of the most efficient. Considering, however, the fact that this is a matter beyond our control; that is, a cause that we can not remove, it is hardly worth while to devote further space, just here, to its consideration. We can not create a new constitution; neither the mischief of a defective inheritance, nor of years of disobedience to the laws of life, can be atoned for—the future only is ours; the balance of vital capital can be expended judiciously, good health regained, often, and life made easy and extended to the utmost limit. Leaving the question of the influence of the spiritual over the physical nature for later consideration (see Conclusion), we have, practically, to take the body as we find it, and aim to conserve its vitality and to improve its condition; and when affected by disease, whether inherited or acquired, to seek its removal by building up the constitution, so to say, by every means in our power.

Notwithstanding the prevalent belief among physicians and laymen to the contrary, a belief based upon the result of a form of treatment as irrational as it is uniform and universal, I agree with Dr. Oswald, who, in his new work—the most entertaining, as well as the soundest health-book extant—asserts that *"Pulmonary consumption,* in its early stages, is perhaps the most curable of all chronic diseases. The records of the dissecting-room prove that in numerous cases lungs, wasted to one-half of their normal size, have been healed, and, after a perfect cicatrization of the tuberculous ulcers, have for years performed all the essential functions of the sound organ.

Still, the actual waste of tissue is never perfectly repaired, and fragmentary lungs, supplying the undiminished wants of the whole organism, must necessarily do double work, and will be less able to respond to the demands of an abnormal exigency.

"But the lungs of a young child of consumptive parents are sound, though very sensitive, and, if the climacteric of the first teens has been passed in safety, or without too serious damage, the problem becomes reduced to the work of preservation and invigoration: the all but intact lungs of the healthy child can be more perfectly redeemed than the rudimentary organs of the far-gone consumptive; the phthisical taint can be more entirely eliminated and the respiratory apparatus strengthened to the degree of becoming the most vigorous part of the organism. The poet Goethe, afflicted in his childhood with spitting of blood and other hectic symptoms, thus completely redeemed himself by a judicious system of self-culture. Chateaubriand, a child of consumptive parents, steeled his constitution by traveling and fasting, and reached his eightieth year.

"By a relapse into imprudent habits, however, the latent spark, which under such circumstances seems to defy the eliminative efforts of half a century, may at any time be fanned into life-consuming flames; but in ninety-nine out of a hundred cases it will be found that the first improvement followed upon a change from a sedentary to an outdoor and active mode of life."[6]

[6] Oswald's "Physical Education."

Anything that constitutes a *tax* upon the system beyond its ability to extract an ultimate good therefrom—for we know that, within certain limits, taxing the powers, the mental, physical and emotional, tends to exalt them—or to put it squarely: anything that overtaxes the system in any direction, tends to induce that state or condition commonly recognized as consumption. No greater error can be made than that of considering this disease as primarily affecting the lungs. The lungs are readily affected by disorder of the digestive organs. While it may not at first be plain to the ordinary reader how catarrh, sore throat, bronchitis and even congestion of the lungs[7] could originate in this manner; it is nevertheless true that they not only can and do thus originate, but this is in fact the most available and constantly operative source of respiratory affections. They may be affected directly by continuity of tissue, or indirectly through the sympathetic system. All understand something about the practical working of the telegraphic system, by which a touch of the wire at Boston, for example, may not only be felt at any point in our own country, but even in England or Europe. How often, in joy or affliction, the wire constitutes a sympathetic connection between friends, families, nations. The nervous system forms a sympathetic connection between the different parts throughout the organism, only it is more complete, ten thousand times over, than the telegraphic or telephonic system. If in these cases the wires were to take on disease,—become inflamed and so affected as to cause the same states, emotions, or disasters, at the point where an unhappy message is received as at the point of departure,—it would constitute for the nation and the world what the sympathetic nervous system does for the animal organism. Should we not, then, deplore its existence, and grieve that we are so "fearfully and wonderfully made"? Nevertheless, it is directly a great boon, and but for this intimate connection between the different portions of the body—for want of this most efficient set of safety valves, so to say—the organs primarily affected would more often become fatally diseased and life speedily terminated. Indeed, in spite of this most wonderful provision of nature, the violations of law are so constant and severe, or so overwhelming upon occasion, that life is often destroyed with but a moment of warning, as in apoplexy, "heart disease," and sunstroke, so called. Strictly speaking, however, even in these cases there have been premonitions without number, dating afar back (see Bright's Disease), which would have prevented the disaster if only they had been known and heeded.

[7] This disorder, which is supposed often to *cause* consumption, is rather a disease of indigestion, and is especially apt to attack patients *already in consumption*, because of their chronically disordered nutritive and respiratory organs.

Says Professor J. C. Zachos (*Studies in Science*):

"... Such is the present system of telegraphing which if it were multiplied so as to include every town and hamlet in the country, yea, even be within the reach of every individual as an operator, would convey but a feeble illustration of the complication, the number, the power, and the perfect unity of a similar system in the human body.

"We have first in each individual cell a galvanic battery. There are countless millions of such cells in the human body, whose united force has never been estimated, but doubtless a million of tons would not approximate to the force they are exerting at any one instant of time. Each of these cells is provided with two nerves; an afferent and an efferent nerve, a carrier to, and a carrier from, that center; each, endowed with different functions by reason of the duality of force generated in each cell: a force of motion and a force of sensation. A number of such cells and nerves may be combined and at a certain point of the circuit they make there, a concentration and accumulation of power by a plexus and convolution of these nerves, around a central substance called 'neureline'—a granulated collection of particles that seem to take the place of the soft iron in the helix, for they are always found in the midst of these convoluted masses of nerves; these masses are called *ganglia*; they are the centers of nervous power and intelligence, connected each with some special group of functions; associated by connecting nerves with each other, and having their central and common connection in the largest ganglion, called the brain.

"No part of the system fails to be visited by these nerves, and although they are not discoverable in every tissue, yet their presence is inferred, because their function is there—sensation or motion, or both.[8]

[8] Is it possible to overestimate the importance of perfect nutrition by which only this wonderful system can be preserved in health? (See "Saline Starvation.")

"We can not at present enter into details in enumerating the number, the structure, the special functions of these several ganglia, which might well be called the telegraphic stations of the body; they vary from the size of a grain of sand, to that of the brain which fills the cavity of the skull.

"But what shall we say of that principle of intelligence which pervades every part of this complicated system; which dwells in each of the thousand millions of cells, where the chemical laboratories are furnishing out of the crude materials of the food, the wonderful organisms of every part of the body? Intelligence and contrivance reign in every cell; combination and co-operation are carried on through the instrumentality of the nervous system. At the centres of co-operation and power there seem to be placed higher forms of intelligence that govern the whole of the subordinate functions by some unitary plan governing thus the functions of the heart, or the liver, or the lungs. Finally, for the moral and social exigencies of man, there is provided an enormous centralization of co-operative intelligences and powers, that seem to have their seat in the brain; but it is a republic and not a monarchy; every individual cell in the body has its representative there, mediately or immediately; every one contributes to the welfare of the whole, and can not be denied its rights, or be neglectful of its duties, without injury, in that proportion, to the whole republic.

"There is a subtle and indefinable health beyond that of the stomach and muscular powers; a man may be torpid in moral brain and intellectual functions, who yet has an excellent appetite and can do the work of an ox.[9] This is not usually regarded as sickness, or needing any physiological treatment. But it is as much so as the grossest form of sickness. A man's temper and disposition may be the only evidence that his liver is out of order. A paroxysm of rage may come from a diseased spleen, and many a murder, arson, and suicide, I doubt not, come from a defective hygiene.

[9] Others, again, are physically as well as mentally impotent, while eating enormously, "the digestion and excretion of superfluous food almost monopolizing the vital energy."

"Physiology is an integral part of theology. Sanitary reforms lie at the foundation of moral reforms. Christianity is health, and the means of escaping from disease.

"No delusion is so vain as to suppose that this world is ever to be Christianized, society purified and exalted, man saved and brought to the divine likeness, while a thousand forms of disease prey upon his vitals, cloud his moral perceptions, enfeeble or exasperate his will, overwhelm him with pain and confusion, even in the midst of his noblest designs; and all this, because he knows not, or respects not sufficiently, the laws of his physical nature; the subtle powers and mechanism of which are as divine in their origin and inflexible in their character as any that govern the soul."

It is not necessary to know, precisely, how this sympathetic or telegraphic system operates in the conservation of health, but all of this knowledge that is essential to us is the understanding of the main fact, to know the nature of a message and from whence it comes, or its probable origin when doubt arises. It is owing to an imperfect knowledge of this law which causes so general a belief in the theory that the internal organism takes on disease readily from the action of cold upon the surface of the body. But, in fact, the skin was especially designed to be played upon by extremes of heat and cold, wind and wet; and human beings are not necessarily such pitiable creatures as they are made to appear from the general supposition that a transient exposure to a current of pure air, whether wet, dry, cold or hot, is likely to bring on disease. "The immediate effects of a displacement of blood from the surface, and its determination to the internal organs, are not," says the *Lancet*, "as was once supposed, sufficient to produce the sort of congestion that issues in inflammation. If it were so, an inflammatory condition would be the common characteristic of our bodily state. When the vascular system is healthy, and that part of the nervous apparatus by which the calibre of the vessels is controlled performs its functions normally, any disturbance of equilibrium in the circulatory system which may have been produced by external cold will be quickly adjusted." Nothing so readily promotes disorder of the vascular system, and of the nervous apparatus which controls it, as to interfere with the nutrition of the nervous system; and in turn, no cause is more effectual, and none more speedy, among the ordinary vicissitudes of life, in depriving the nerves and tissues of their appropriate aliment, than an excessive or otherwise unwholesome diet and the consequent disturbance of the organs of nutrition; and the excess is increased relatively, and the disorder intensified, in proportion as the body is sweltered with clothing and defrauded of the "breath of life"—outdoor air. It is a very significant comment on the cold-air fallacy, that people of all ages, sexes, occupations and social positions, and in all conditions of *general* health, catch cold, say to-day, from the slightest exposures, often, indeed, they are totally at a loss to account for them except upon one surmise or another, like that of the old lady who "caught her death o' cold *taking gruel out of a damp basin*"; while next month, or next week, perhaps, the same individuals endure the most extreme exposure, as, for example, riding for hours in face of a driving rain or snow-storm, until wet and chilled through and through; or, perhaps, being turned out at night in bitter cold, half clad, to find their way from their burning dwelling to a distant neighbor's—in short, they may suffer the most taxing exposures and yet "catch" nothing more than a good appetite for a warm dinner or a cheery fireside. The boy who, as was supposed, caught a fearful cold one warm day last week, from merely stepping to the door bareheaded, stole away yesterday, when the *mercury* was *twenty or thirty degrees lower*, and bareheaded and barefooted, paddled in the frog-pond until his clothes were wet through and his lips blue with cold, and yet he turned out this morning without a trace of disease! Can we learn nothing from constantly occurring instances of this character? The simple fact is, in such cases, in the first instance the victims were in bad condition, they had found the end of their rope, so to say, *i.e.*, they had reached a point where from continued bad living the system could no longer contain the accumulated impurities and the overflow had to come, and come it would, sooner or later (and the later, the more severe), without even the influence of the slightest current of air, or any form of exposure. If a slight chill was experienced it arose from the internal fever, and not, as was foolishly supposed, from the puff of pure air that was felt *co-incidently*. But in the second instance, the "cold" of last week had *cleansed the system* more or less completely, and now, owing to the improved condition, the really severe exposures give rise to no symptoms of disease—the temporary inconvenience from the wet or the cold is all.

Personally, I have been a life-long sufferer from colds, and as with every one (how many pass a year without "a cold" of some sort?) they came in a variety of forms, from the "snuffles" of crammed infancy and the "hay fever" of adult age, to neuralgia, rheumatism, and the like. No matter what name may be settled on, finally, to describe the disease, whether rheumatism, neuralgia, sick headache, kidney complaint, bilious fever, or what not, the victim is sure to say: "I caught a severe cold some way, and it settled"—wherever the uneasy symptoms are felt.[10] "A succession of colds" is the commonly-named *excuse*, and the honestly-believed-in *cause* of lung affections, including consumption; but as the phrase is usually understood, it is the veriest blunder—the most pernicious blunder possible. Hence the space devoted to this subject. Some years ago I made a change in my habits as to diet and clothing: I quite abruptly abandoned the use of heavy-weight garments, heavy flannels, and the practice of "bundling up" upon occasions of exposure, and I gave up the three-meal system, and the fish, flesh, and fowl, and most of the accompaniments of the flesh diet, and have since lived mainly on vegetable food. I eat twice a day, nominally, but invariably skip a meal if there is any sign of indigestion, or whenever I think I should be better off without eating. I eat on an average about a dozen meals a week, each less in amount, though more nutritious than formerly. This keeps my appetite always perfect, but I am never "hungry," as when I ate three meals every day, "work or play."

[10] And so with non-healing wounds, cuts, bruises, "cold-sores," etc. Those people who have their bodies built up of impure material, who are unsound through and through, always "catch cold in it" when they have a wound of any kind or a sore; and their flesh is easily wounded and sores come often, more or less mysteriously, and the most trifling wound that would, in the case of a healthy man, woman, or child, heal readily, and in a few days be entirely well, in their case "festers," and may be troublesome for weeks or months, perhaps necessitating the amputation of a finger, hand, or a limb, or even causing death. Healthy people have no occasion for sores, boils, etc; but if filth exists in the system, these little volcanoes tend to eliminate it, and to the prevention of other diseases. The suppression of catarrhal or diarrhœal discharges often results in dangerous sicknesses, even fatal sicknesses, unless their cause is first removed. (See Bright's Disease.)

I was formerly hungry before every meal, and if any one of them was delayed for a single hour there was sure to be a faint and languid feeling—a disinclination for, and a seeming inability to, labor—which, however, would usually disappear if I kept on working! From this I finally learned a most valuable lesson, viz: that the craving appetite that tempts one to forestall the regular meal hour is a species of "poison-hunger," akin to that which torments the inebriate if his customary dram is not forthcoming. In either case, whether the congested stomach *seems* to crave solid or liquid stimulants, the only wise thing is to abstain, remove or relieve the inflammatory state of the stomach by giving it rest from digestive labor, and by judicious drinking of pure water, and then eat and drink so as to prevent a recurrence of the disorder. So universal is this disagreeable feeling with three-meal-flesh-and-pastry eaters and coffee-drinkers that Marshall Hall, evidently himself ignorant of its nature and cause, refers what he styles the "temper disease" to the *mauvais quart d'heure* before dinner!

Since adopting the new plan I can truly say that when I live up to it, as do most of the time, I *never* have any of the symptoms of what is commonly known as cold, nor, indeed, any kind of physical inconvenience whatever. And yet, only twelve years ago, my physical condition was such that I bade fair to follow my mother, an aunt, an uncle, a sister, and a brother, all of whom died of tubercular consumption under the prevailing general regimen and medical treatment, both of which I design in this treatise to unqualifiedly denounce.

In order, however, to see if I could, by exposure, cause the well-known symptoms of cold, I have made many experiments, some of which I will name: I have walked in snow and slop with low shoes until both shoes and socks were soaked through, and have sat thus for an hour or more; after wearing all-wool flannels during moderate weather, I have, upon the approach of *colder weather*, removed my under-garments, and have then attended to my outdoor affairs, minus the overcoat habitually worn; I have slept in winter in a current blowing directly about my head and shoulders; upon going to bed, I have sat in a strong current, *entirely nude*, for a quarter of an hour, on a very cold, damp night in the fall of the year; I have worn a flannel gown, and slept under heavy-weight bed-covers one night, and in cotton night-shirt and light-weight bed-clothes the next. These and similar experiments I have made repeatedly, and have never been able to catch cold. I become cold, sometimes quite cold, and become warm again, that is all. On the other hand, changing the form of my experiments, returning to my old way, the prevalent style of living—a "generous diet" and a full meal every five or six hours through the day—I have found no difficulty in *accumulating* a cold; and within a reasonable length of time could count upon it, although, now, a part of the programme consisted in taking the most extreme care to avoid what are commonly reckoned as exposures—keeping my feet ever warm and dry, paying strict attention to wraps,[11] etc. This is not simply my own individual experience, but, also, of others who, either of their own accord or through my suggestion, have carefully studied the matter; while rational hygienists, generally, attest to the main fact, that they endure all the ordinary vicissitudes of life without often being troubled with this most disagreeable complaint.

[11] Said an observing friend to me: "I am apt to catch cold when I *put on* my winter flannels; why is that?" With those who may happen to be already near the brink, this effect is likely to follow the addition of an extra layer of flannel to the ordinary dress, unless they leave out a layer of food, so to say, or the weather happens to be enough colder on that day, to counteract the extra clothing.

In the course of my experimentation, whenever I have fed my cold as far as I wished or dared to go, I have, in every instance, banished the disease by abstaining from food and indulging in extra rations of outdoor air—rain or shine. I have never known this remedy to fail of "breaking up" a common cold in twenty-four to forty-eight hours, whatever the age, sex, or occupation of the individual, and regardless of the supposed origin of the disease. Of course the size of the "dose" must bear some relation to the severity of the disorder. Whenever I have chosen to prolong one of these experiments by continuing to eat heartily, as is customary with people in general, I have found my experience identical with that of others: the symptoms would increase in severity, and to acute catarrh, headache, slight feverishness, and languor, would be added sore throat, perhaps, with pressure at the lungs, hoarseness, increased fever, and entire indisposition for exertion. In this case two, perhaps three, days' fasting (one, maybe two, in bed) would be required, with a little extra sponging of the skin, to reduce the fever and completely restore the balance. I have, to be sure, never been reckless enough to subject my system to the influence of impure air—to the quality of air, for example, that is the daily and nightly reliance of ninety and nine families in the hundred, rich or poor, in the city or country—this I would never do; and for this reason my "colds" would be less severe, other things equal, than those of my neighbors, and more readily amenable to "treatment"; but the principle holds good in all cases. There are all degrees of obtuseness observable in the mental efforts of our fellow-creatures: I have had persons reply to this, that they "couldn't agree" with me entirely in my position, for they had "tried the remedy," when, in fact, as they would more or less hesitatingly admit, they had kept up their three-meal feeding, even after the appetite had passed the craving stage and the fitful stage; and even after food became loathsome they had punished themselves more or less *gruelly*; but, finally, driven to the wall, and eating little or nothing for a few days or weeks, because it was physically impossible to eat more, they have the assurance to declare, or the sublime stupidity to believe, that they have tried the fasting-cure, and that while "it might cure some," it wouldn't answer for them! And they usually add—of all aphorisms the most foolish and misleading—"one's meat, another's poison."[12] It results, in such cases, that, if the individual recovers, he does so as the effect of seven-eighths starvation, involuntarily practiced, and extending over a period of weeks or months, when a few days of total abstinence early enough in the contest, before the appetite declined, would have saved the system from the depletion of a long-continued strain.

[12] Were I to summarize the arguments against the saying, that "what is meat for one is poison for another," I would put it something like this: Its author, and the people, have been deceived in that one person can *bear* what another can not. Some constitutions have withstood the worst habits—violations of all the known laws of life—gluttony, intemperance to the degree of almost constant drunkenness, the grossest and most constant immorality in departments the most exhausting, until passed what we call old age—and still have rounded out a full century of life. Many, on the other hand, of frailer make, have, by reason of a tithe of such misconduct, been swept into premature graves, at middle-age, early manhood, or even in youth. Others, again, like the last named, and rapidly following them to destruction, have been kept back, put on the mending hand, and have lived fairly long lives, from renouncing their immoral practices, or, perhaps, simply their "unhealthy" practices as to diet, when these have been their only faults. As elsewhere remarked, thousands of lives have been saved and robust health regained, or gained for the first time, from adopting the vegetarian, as against the prevailing "mixed," diet. I believe that the reverse of this will not be even claimed by any one who has a *right* to claim expert knowledge. It may be relied upon that no substance that is positively wholesome for one person, is, *in and of itself*, injurious—speaking with relation to food. To this rule, it must be admitted, there are a few, isolated and, as yet, not fully explained exceptions—but the rule holds good; and it is equally certain that whatever is, *in and of itself*, harmful for one person to eat or drink, smoke, snuff, or chew, whether animal, vegetable, or mineral, food or medicine, is not good, certainly not *best*, for any other person to eat, drink, absorb, or take into the system in any manner. It is true that there are many things transpiring before our eyes

every day which, to the superficial observer—and only the well-informed upon a given subject can see beneath the surface—form apparent exceptions to this rule—even to the degree of seeming to cast it aside as not a rule; nevertheless, no rule holds more uniformly true than this.

Lest it be inferred that I design to intimate that any one could at once imitate my cold air experiments with impunity, immediately upon changing his method of living, I hasten to say that not all could do this, any more than they could imitate the muscular feats of an athlete. As the depraved muscular system has to be built up by degrees and by long practice, so the life-long sweltered skin can become accustomed to extreme changes of temperature only by a somewhat gradual change of habit. Besides, it takes some time for the general system to come under the influence of a pure diet; and, again, the best of remedies have to be graduated in amount to the present condition of the patient. However, I am sure that most persons who will accustom themselves to an out-door life and to light clothing, have only to reform their eating-habits to make themselves virtually disease proof; while *all* classes may derive great benefit from a rational application of the principle.

That certain symptoms, popularly called cold, are often *excited* by exposure to fresh air, damp air, draughts, and the like, is true enough; and we should be devoutly thankful for this provision of Nature. But it is likewise true that these "exposures" do not, and can not, *originate* the disease that *in its exit* manifests the well-known symptoms. *That* already exists, and has been for months, perhaps, accumulating in the system; and now, an unusual amount of fresh air in the lungs and in contact with the skin, has so *invigorated the organism* as to enable it to institute measures for thrusting out the real disease; hence catarrh, cough, expectoration, *fever*—for the name, cold, is a complete misnomer, and based upon a misconception as to the real nature of the disorder: the patient may be never so chilly, but the thermometer placed under the tongue at once shows that the temperature is above the normal standard. Says Dr. Oswald:[13] "Rightly interpreted, the external symptoms of disease constitute a restorative process that can not be brought to a satisfactory issue till the cause of the evil is removed. So that, in fact, the air-hater confounds the cause of his recovery with the cause of his disease. Among nations who pass their lives out-doors, catarrh and scrofula are unknown; not fresh air, but the want of it, is the cause of countless diseases, of fatal diseases where people are in the habit of *nailing down* their windows every winter to keep their children from opening them. The only objection to a 'draught' through a defective window is, that the draught is generally not strong enough. An influx of fresh air into a sick-room is a ray of light into darkness, a messenger of Vishnu visiting an abode of the damned. Cold air," he continues, "is a disinfectant, and under the pressure of a high wind a modicum of oxygen will penetrate a house in spite of closed windows. This circumstance alone has preserved the lives of thousands whom no cough syrup, or cod-liver oil could have saved."

[13] "Physical Education," by F. L. Oswald. M.D. New York: D. Appleton & Co.

Referring once more to the sympathetic telegraph, we find, for instance, that a small wound in the foot may produce lock-jaw; a blow on the elbow makes the fingers tingle; touch the soft palate with the finger and the stomach offers up its contents; and in the same manner, substantially, irritation or congestion of the stomach or intestines will give rise to tickling in the throat, itching of the nose,[14] etc., etc.; and if the primary disease be severe or constant, or of frequent occurrence, acute or chronic disease of the lungs may result. Indeed, I am led to the conclusion that the lungs seldom become disordered in any other manner. The pneumogastric nerve with its various branches forms a close "sympathy" between the brain and the larynx, bronchi, lungs, liver, heart and stomach. Is there, in reason and common sense, any necessity for argument to prove that of all the organs the stomach is the most abused; or rather, that of all our abuses of this wonderful temple of the body those inflicted by the medium of the alimentary system are the most flagrant and most constant?

[14] It is not from *habit,* simply, that children pick the nose, and half the occupants of a drawing-room car, even, devote a sly moment to the same inspiring occupation! Observe the prevalence of red noses, enlarged nostrils, etc., among coffee drinkers and dyspeptics, as well as liquor drinkers.

Consider for one moment that the food taken from day to day should be plain and simple, and that in quality and quantity it should bear a close relation to the following circumstances or conditions, viz.: (1) to the season and the climate; (2) to the purity of the air habitually breathed; (3) amount of clothing worn; (4) amount of mental and physical labor performed; (5) the existing physical condition as to (*a*) appetite—whether normal or abnormal, as for example, ravenous, fitful or none at all; (*b*) strength—whether full, or exhausted from fatigue: (6) mental state—whether the mind is at ease, or from one or another cause distressed, as with grief, anger,[15] etc.; (7) the natural constitution—whether delicate or robust. How many, let me ask, in any community consider *any* of these conditions, or are to any extent influenced by them? Not that the question is, after all, as complicated as would at first sight appear; on the contrary, it is very simple, indeed. We have only to clothe ourselves in loose and comfortable garments; keep clean; breathe out-door air—whether we are indoors or out, day and night; [16] lead an active, useful life, rest when tired, never eat without a good relish, nor, as a rule, when there is "gnawing" at the stomach, nor when the body is exhausted with fatigue or the mind in a badly disturbed state. Eat but twice daily and of the simplest and purest food, *i.e.*, the cereal grains, vegetables and fruits. Ordinarily, a little animal food—unaccompanied by greasy or stimulating condiments—will not affect a robust person seriously; but it is not essential to health, speaking generally, and in depraved conditions of the system it may be set down as detrimental; although lean beef or mutton, plainly cooked, and served without "seasoning," is doubtless preferable to bolted flour or impoverished vegetables, whose dissipated salts are mistakenly supposed to be "restored" in the form of artificial salt (see "Saline Starvation.")

[15] Few causes are more readily promotive of indigestion than the indulgence of such emotions, and none presents a greater obstacle to the recovery of a consumptive patient than the habitual subjection of the mind to unhappy reflections of whatsoever character. It is especially important for both patient and all who approach him to avoid, so far as possible, every disquieting influence.

[16] "Azotized air affects the lungs as the substitution of excrements for nourishing food would affect our digestive organs: corruption sets in; pulmonary phthisis is, in fact, a process of putrefaction.

"No ventilatory contrivance can compare with the simple plan of opening a window; in wet nights a 'rain-shutter' (a blind with large, overlapping bars) will keep a room both airy and dry. In every bedroom, one of the upper windows should be kept open night and day, except in storms, accompanied with rain or with a degree of cold exceeding 10° Fahr. In warm summer nights open every window in the house and every door connecting the bedroom with the adjoining apartments. Create a thorough draught. Before we can hope to fight consumption with any chance of success, we have to get rid of the *night-air superstition*. Like the dread of cold water, raw fruit, etc., it is founded on that mistrust of our instincts which we owe to our anti-natural religion. It is probably the most prolific single cause of impaired health, even among the civilized nations of our enlightened age, though its absurdity rivals the grossest delusions of the witchcraft era. The subjection of holy reason to hearsays could hardly go further.

"'Beware of the night-wind; be sure and close your windows after dark!' In other words, beware of God's free air; be sure and infect your lungs with the stagnant, azotized, and offensive atmosphere of your bedroom. In other words, beware of the rock spring; stick to sewerage. Is night-air injurious? Is there a single tenable pretext for such an idea? Since the day of creation that air has been breathed with impunity by millions of different animals—tender, delicate creatures, some of them—fawns, lambs, and young birds. The moist night-air of the tropical forests is breathed with impunity by our next relatives, the anthropoid apes—the same apes that soon perish with consumption in the close though generally well-warmed atmosphere of our northern menageries. Thousands of soldiers, hunters, and lumbermen sleep every night in tents and open sheds without the least injurious consequences; men in the last stage of consumption have recovered by adopting a semi-savage mode of life, and camping out-doors in all but the stormiest nights. Is it the draught you fear, or the contrast of temperature? Blacksmiths and railroad-conductors seem to thrive under such influences. Draught? Have you never seen boys skating in the teeth of a snow-storm at the rate of fifteen miles an hour? 'They counteract the effects of the cold air by vigorous exercise.' Is there no other way of keeping warm? Does the north wind damage the fine lady sitting motionless in her sleigh, or the pilot and helmsman of a storm-tossed vessel? It can not be the *inclemency* of the open air, for, even in sweltering summer nights, the sweet south wind, blessed by all creatures that draw the breath of life, brings no relief to the victim of aërophobia. There is no doubt that families who have freed themselves from the curse of that superstition can live out and out healthier in the heart of a great city than its slaves on the airiest highland of the southern Apennines."—("Physical Education.")

CHAPTER III.

CONSUMPTION—(*Continued*).

The country boor says he must have meat to make muscle; and all the while his vegetarian team is twitching him and his plow along the furrow. Where does he suppose they get their muscles?—THOREAU.

Stupidly ignorant, or unmindful, of the fact that there are, in this country and Europe, hundreds of thousands of people of all ages, sexes and social positions, who live year in and year out mainly, and a large proportion strictly, on the vegetarian diet, and live in health, not only, but found perfect health by abandoning the common mixed diet and coming nearer to first principles—notwithstanding all this, still the farce goes on among the scientists of "proving" by chemical analyses, pretty theories and specious arguments, that man "can not subsist in health on a vegetarian diet."[17]

[17] Jules Virey estimates that four-tenths of the human race subsist exclusively on a vegetable diet, and that seven-tenths are practically (though not on principle) vegetarians. Virchow estimates the total number at eighty-five per cent.—OSWALD.

"The matter is this: in a cold climate we can not thrive without a modicum of fat, but that fat need not come from slaughtered animals. In a colder country than England, the East-Russian peasant, remarkable for his robust health and longevity, subsists on cabbage-soup, rye-bread, and vegetable oils. In a colder country than England, the Gothenburg shepherds live chiefly on milk, barley bread, and esculent roots. The strongest men of the three manliest races of the present world are non-carnivorous: the Turanian mountaineers of Daghestan and Lesghia, the Mandingo tribes of

Senegambia, and the Schleswig-Holstein *Bauern*, who furnish the heaviest cuirassiers for the Prussian army and the ablest seamen for the Hamburg navy. Nor is it true that flesh is an indispensable, or even the best, brain-food. Pythagoras, Plato, Seneca, Paracelsus, Spinoza, Peter Bayle, and Shelley were vegetarians; so were Franklin and Lord Byron in their best years. Newton, while engaged in writing his 'Principia' and 'Quadrature of Curves,' abstained entirely from animal food, which he had found by experience to be unpropitious to severe mental application. The ablest modern physiologists incline to the same opinion. 'I use animal food because I have not the opportunity to choose my diet,' says Professor Welch, of Yale; 'but, whenever I have abstained from it, I have found my health mentally, morally, and physically better.'"—("Physical Education.")

With regard to the muscular vigor of vegetarians: if they have not become noted as "winners of rowing, walking, or boxing matches," it is chiefly because they are rarely sporting men; besides, they are as yet in this country—although their numbers are quite rapidly increasing—in a very small minority; but, of late, since this objection has been so frequently raised, vegetarians have entered the lists, notably in England, in bicycle races, and have distanced their meat-eating rivals in long races, showing greater staying powers.

Says the London *Lancet*: "In the summer of 1872, it became necessary to shift the rails on upwards of 500 miles of permanent way on the Great Western line, from the broad to the narrow gauge, and there was only a fortnight to do it in. The work to be got through was enormous. About 3,000 men were employed, and they worked double time, sometimes from four in the morning till nine at night. Not a soul was sick, sorry, or drunk, and the work was accomplished on time. What was the extraordinary support of this wonderful spurt of muscular strength and energy? Weak oatmeal gruel. There was no beer, spirits, or alcoholic drink in any form. Here," continues the *Lancet,* "is a very old and well-known agent, cheap enough, and easily procured, capable of imparting 'staying power' better, probably, than anything else, which is not employed to anything like the extent it might be with advantage."

The principal part of the ration allowed in the above case was one and one-half pounds of oatmeal. In view of the immense labor performed by these men on that quantity of this cereal, can it be wondered at that the sedentary dyspeptic who essays to "diet" on three full meals of such food comes to grief? For him a single moderate meal of grain food, with fruit, would be a generous ration.

To very many the term "vegetarian" seems almost to imply one who is restricted to a diet of turnips and water. But Epicurus, the god of gluttons, was himself a vegetarian, for while he regarded pleasure as the *summum bonum*, and placed the pleasures of the table first, still, he knew that a simple fare was most conducive to health and comfort in this life. As to variety: "with five kinds of cereals, three legumina, eight species of esculent roots, ten or twelve nutritive herbs, thirty to forty varieties of tree fruits, besides berries and nuts, a vegetarian might emulate the Duc de Polignac, who refused to eat the same dish more than once per season."

In view of the constant violations of natural law as to quality, quantity and frequency of meals, I would say that it is from the nature of the case impossible for people living in the prevailing manner to avoid digestive disorders;[18] in practice I find *none* altogether exempt from them, except the very small class of abstemious vegetarians referred to—an individual or a family, or two, in each community—all others are more or less dyspeptic, and *dyspepsia* is *incipient consumption*. Thousands of dyspeptics are oblivious as to the true nature of their disorder, simply because the most marked symptoms in their cases, *now*, are affections of the throat and lungs. The popular ignorance in this direction amply accounts for the appalling fact that respiratory diseases destroy the lives of about one-third, and consumption alone one-fifth of all who die in this country. When dyspepsia has blossomed into consumption, unless the primary disease—that of the stomach and intestines—is removed—an impossibility except by a radical change from the evil dietetic habits that have caused it—nature is powerless to heal the lungs, because (1) the inflammation is being perpetually propagated, and (2) the entire nutritive system is becoming more and more hopelessly diseased.

[18] "I think I shall not be far wrong if I say that there are few subjects more important to the well-being of man than the selection and preparation of his food. Our forefathers in their wisdom have provided, by ample and generously endowed organizations, for the dissemination of moral precepts in relation to human conduct, and for the constant supply of sustenance to meet the cravings of religious emotions common to all sorts and conditions of men. In these provisions no student of human nature can fail to recognize the spirit of wisdom and a lofty purpose. But it is not a sign of ancestral wisdom that so little thought has been bestowed on the teaching of what we should eat and drink; that the relations, not only between food and a healthy population, but between food and virtue, between the process of digestion and the state of mind which results from it, have occupied a subordinate place in the practical arrangements of life. No doubt there has long been some practical acknowledgment, on the part of a few educated persons, of the simple fact that a man's temper, and consequently many of his actions, depends on such an alternative as whether he habitually digests his food well or ill; whether the meals which he eats are properly converted into healthy material, suitable for the ceaseless work of building up both muscle and brain; or whether unhealthy products constantly pollute the course of nutritive supply. But the truth of that fact has never been generally admitted to an extent at all comparable with its exceeding importance. It produces no practical result on the habits of men in the least degree commensurate with the pregnant import it contains. For it is certain that an adequate recognition of the value of proper food to the individual in maintaining a high standard of health, in prolonging healthy life (the prolongation of unhealthy life being small gain either to the individual or to the community), and thus largely promoting cheerful temper, prevalent good-nature, and improved moral tone, would require almost a revolution in the habits of a large part of the community.

"The general outlines of a man's mental character and physical tendencies are doubtless largely determined by the impress of race and family. That is, the scheme of the building, its characteristics and dimensions, are inherited; but to a very large extent the materials and filling in of the framework depend upon his food and training. By the latter term may be understood all that relates to mental and moral and even to physical education, in part already assumed to be fairly provided for, and therefore not further to be considered here. No matter, then, how consummate the scheme of the architect, nor how vast the design, more or less of failure to rear the edifice results when the materials are ill chosen or wholly unworthy to be used. Many other sources of failure there may be which it is no part of my business to note; but the influence of food is not only itself cardinal in rank, but, by priority of action, gives rise to other and secondary agencies.

"The slightest sketch of the commonest types of human life will suffice to illustrate this truth.

"To commence, I fear it must be admitted that the majority of infants are reared on imperfect milk by weak or ill-fed mothers. And thus it follows that the signs of disease, of feeble vitality, or of fretful disposition, may be observed at a very early age, and are apparent in symptoms of indigestion or in the cravings of want manifested by the 'peevish' and sleepless infant. In circumstances where there is no want of abundant nutriment, over-feeding or complicated forms of food, suitable only for older persons, produce for this infant troubles which are no less grave than those of the former. In the next stage of life, among the poor the child takes his place at the parents' table, where lack of means, as well as of knowledge, deprives him of food more suitable than the rough fare of the adult.... On the whole, perhaps he is not much worse off than the child of the well-to-do, who becomes a pet, and is already familiarized with complex and too solid forms of food and stimulating drinks which custom and self-indulgence have placed on the daily table. And soon afterward commence in consequence—and entirely in consequence, a fact it is impossible too much to emphasize—the 'sick-headaches' and 'bilious attacks,' which pursue their victim through half a lifetime, to be exchanged for gout or worse at or before the grand climacteric. And so common are these evils that they are regarded by people in general as a necessary appanage of 'poor humanity.' No notion can be more erroneous, since it is absolutely true that the complaints referred to are self-engendered, form no necessary part of our physical nature, and for their existence are dependent almost entirely on our habits in relation to food and drink. I except, of course, those cases in which hereditary tendencies are so strong as to produce these evils, despite some care on the part of the unfortunate victim of an ancestor's self-indulgence. Equally, however, on the part of that little-to-be-revered progenitor was ill-chosen food, or more probably excess in quantity, the cause of disease, and not the physical nature of man.

"The next stage of boyhood transfers the child just spoken of to a public school, where too often inappropriate diet, at the most critical period of growth, has to be supplemented from other sources. It is almost unnecessary to say that chief among these are the pastry-cook and the vender of portable provisions, for much of which latter that skin-stuffed compound of unknown origin, an uncertified sausage, may be accepted as the type.

"After this period arise the temptations to drink, among the youth of all classes, whether at beer-house, tavern, or club. For it is often taught in the bosom of the family, by the father's example and by the mother's precept, that wine, beer, and spirits are useful, nay, necessary to health, and that they augment the strength. And the lessons thus inculcated and too well learned were but steps which led to wider experience in the pursuit of health and strength by larger use of the same means. Under such circumstances it often happens, as the youth grows up, that a flagging appetite or a failing digestion habitually demands a dram before or between meals, and that these are regarded rather as occasions to indulge in variety of liquor than as repasts for nourishing the body. It is not surprising, with such training, that the true object of both eating and drinking is entirely lost sight of. The gratification of acquired tastes usurps the function of that zest which healthy appetite produces; and the intention that food should be adapted to the physical needs of the body and the healthy action of the mind is forgotten altogether. So it often comes to pass that at middle age, when man finds himself in the full current of life's occupations, struggling for pre-eminence with his fellows, indigestion has become persistent in some of its numerous forms, shortens his 'staying power,' or spoils his judgment or temper. And, besides all this, few causes are more potent than an incompetent stomach to engender habits of selfishness and egotism. A constant care to provide little personal wants of various kinds, thus rendered necessary, cultivates these sentiments, and they influence the man's whole character in consequence."

"But it is necessary to say at this point, and I desire to say it emphatically, that the subject of food need not, even with the views just enunciated, be treated in an ascetic spirit. It is to be considered in relation to a principle, in which we may certainly believe, that aliments most adapted to develop the individual, sound in body and mind, shall not only be most acceptable but that they may be selected and prepared so as to afford scope for the exercise of a refined taste, and produce a fair degree of that pleasure naturally associated with the function of the palate, and derived from a study of the table. For it is certain that nine-tenths of the gormandism which is practiced—for the most part a matter of faith without knowledge—is no more a source of gratification to the eater's gustatory sense than it is of digestible sustenance to his body."—"FOOD AND FEEDING," by Sir Henry Thompson.

The stomach, more especially after long years of abusive treatment, is one of the least sensitive organs. "If it had nerves as sensitive as our finger-tips, our attention would be so much taken up with the ordinary digestion of food that we could not properly attend to our work or studies." At first, in infancy, it is more sensitive, and any excess of food is thrown off, but ere many months the disorder grows worse and deeper-seated, and in the course of years stomachs become so diseased as to give no sign, except when unusually outraged. It may have sores without knowing it. Dr. Beaumont saw sores in St. Martin's stomach after the latter had drunk liquor, but they occasioned no pain. "Cold sores," chapped lips, parched or pimpled tongue or mouth, furred tongue, etc., etc., are but signs of serious disease of the stomach and intestines, and, consequently, of the entire organism.

I have classed as one of the most natural and effective measures for the preservation of health or the cure of disease, *rest*; for diseased organs, rest[19] and light tasks; for the healthy person who desires to keep well, I have said, "rest when tired." Unfortunately many people, and more especially consumptives, never know when they are tired, but work habitually, until they are exhausted. With the latter, this is usually set down to willfulness or lack of judgment. "She won't listen to reason," says the anxious husband. "She is always overdoing," says another. Jockeys, describing horses thus affected, call them "pullers": it is the same disease—indigestion. Reason being dethroned by the poisoned circulation in the brain, Nature, through muscular action, essays to excrete the toxic elements. This is *stimulation* (see "Coffee.")

[19] The various excretory organs, as the bowels, kidneys, liver, as well as the digestive apparatus, are relieved by fasting, or diminishing the food ration.

It is the stimulus imparted by the thrice daily ingestion of so many unnatural and indigestible articles that compose the mixed diet, which prevents so many from resting when they are tired. With others, however, the effect is quite the reverse: some are always complaining of a "tired feeling." There is a genuine lack of vital force occasioned by lack of nourishment. When this feeling is experienced on rising, it is usually, almost invariably, at least in part, the effect of close sleeping-rooms. Many persons,—some who are fat, and called healthy, others, perhaps, lean,—are called "lazy" who are positively weak, too weak to work without great effort such as lookers-on know nothing about, although most people may have had similar feelings occasionally—the "after-dinner laziness." This special form of disease has previously been spoken of. (See p. 34).

Nutrition is the grand factor in the prevention or cure of disease. It may be said, truly enough, that the blood-*aerating* capacity remains throughout equal, often superior, to the blood-*making* capacity; and consumption may be appropriately described as *dyspeptic starvation*. (See "Saline Starvation.") In those instances where the capital stock (of vitality) is exhausted the victims of this disease must die; but thousands of cases pronounced after a long course of medication and stimulation, hopeless, have been restored by a simple diet and an out-door life. Even hygienic institutes have failed to apply this principle in its entirety when brought face to face with cases that demanded "heroic treatment;" influenced in some measure, possibly, by the popular distrust of their methods, especially the deep prejudice against a restricted diet—now, however, rapidly disappearing—they have hitherto erred continually on the side of excess. Nevertheless, they restore to health, or greatly benefit, ninety per cent. of the broken down invalids who come to them, usually, as a last resort.

I desire here to note particularly the change now going on in the minds of the most eminent and practical physicians in this and European countries, concerning the use of beef-tea. It is found by chemical analysis to be almost identical with "chamber-lye"—the favorite prescription of our grandmothers—and although more agreeable to the taste than urine, even when the latter is drowned in treacle, it is, in my opinion, always injurious, especially in sickness, when, of course, the excretory system is already taxed to the utmost. Most people, even in health, have more than they can well do to excrete their own, once, without swallowing any portion of the waste of animals!

Says Dr. Brunton:

"We find only too frequently that both doctors and patients think that the strength is sure to be kept up if a sufficient quantity of beef-tea can only be got down; but I think it a question whether beef-tea may not very frequently (?) be actually injurious, and whether the products of muscular waste which constitute the chief portion of beef-tea, beef-essence, or even the beef itself, may not, under certain circumstances, be actually poisonous."

"In many cases of nervous depression we find a feeling of weakness and prostration coming on during digestion, and becoming so very marked about the second hour after a meal has been taken, and at the very time when absorption is going on, that we can hardly do otherwise than ascribe it to actual poisoning by digestive products absorbed into the circulation. From the observation of a number of cases, I came to the conclusion that the languor and faintness of which many patients complained, and which occurred about eleven and four o'clock, was due to actual poisoning by the products of digestion of breakfast and lunch; but at the time when I arrived at this conclusion I had no experimental data to show that the products of digestion were actually poisonous in themselves; and only within the last few months have I seen the conclusions to which I had arrived by clinical observation, confirmed by experiments made in the laboratory. Such experiments have been made by Professor Albertoni, of Genoa, and by Dr. Schmidt-Mühlheim, in Professor Ludwig's laboratory at Leipsic."

"Professor Albertoni and Dr. Schmidt-Mühlheim independently made the discovery that peptones prevented the coagulation of the blood in dogs, and the latter, under Ludwig's direction, has also investigated their action upon the circulation. He finds that, when injected into a vein, they greatly depress the circulation, so that the blood-pressure falls very considerably; and when the quantity injected is large, they produce a soporose condition, complete arrest of the secretion by the kidneys,[20] convulsions, and death. From these experiments it is evident that the normal products of digestion are poisons of no inconsiderable power, and that if they reach the general circulation in large quantities they may produce very alarming, if not dangerous symptoms."

[20] See "Bright's Disease."

"Instead of trying to keep up the strength, as it is termed, by loading the stomach with food, the exhausted brain-worker should rather lean toward abstinence from food, and especially toward abstinence from alcoholic liquors.[21] The feeling of muscular weakness and lassitude, which I have already had occasion to mention as frequently coming on about two hours after meals, is not uncommonly met with in persons belonging to the upper classes who are well fed and have little exercise. It is perhaps seen in its most marked form in young women or girls who have left school, and who, having no definite occupation in life, are indisposed to any exercise, either bodily or mental. I am led to look upon this condition as one of poisoning, both on account of the time of its occurrence, during the absorption of digestive products, and by reason of the peculiar symptoms—viz., a curious weight in the legs and arms, the patient describing them as feeling like lumps of lead. These symptoms so much resemble the effect which would be produced by a poison like curare, that one could hardly help attributing them to the action of a depressant or paralyzer of motor nerves or centers. The recent researches of Ludwig and Schmidt-Mühlheim render it exceedingly probable that peptones are the poisonous agents in these cases; and an observation which I have made seems to confirm this conclusion, for I found that the weakness and languor were less after meals consisting of farinaceous food only. My observations, however, are not sufficiently extensive to absolutely convince me that they are entirely absent after meals of this sort, so that possibly the poisoning by peptones, although one cause of the languor, is not to be looked upon as the only cause."[22]

[21] See chapter on Coffee.

[22] "Indigestion as a Cause of Nervous Depression." By T. Lauder Brunton. M.D., F.R.S., in *Practitioner*.

I am able to vouch for a number of cases of consumption, and marasmus, in which, under tonic treatment and frequent meals, the patients were steadily declining, but which yielded, finally, to the influence of the one-meal-a-day system: comparative rest of the diseased alimentary organs, and consequent improvement in the digestive and assimilative functions proved the needed "stimulant." The Boston *Journal of Chemistry*, of February, 1882, gives the history of a well-authenticated case, of an old man of 70 years, who had been declining with pulmonary consumption for three years, and who was pronounced incurable, who was made convalescent by a voluntary and absolute fast of 43 days—taking water freely, however, during the time—and, following this with the "bread and fruit" diet, was restored to health.

Let us contrast this method of *restoring* the nutritive organs with that of "curing" them by medication:

J. Milner Fothergill, M.D., truly says (in the *Practitioner*), that "it is more important to study the tongue than to go over the chest with a stethoscope, and that attention to the stomach and bowels is just as essential as the treatment of night sweats. When the tongue is covered with thick fur it is nearly or quite useless to give iron or cod-liver oil; for the tongue is the indicator of the state of the intestinal canal, and absorption through the thick layer of dead epithelial cells is impossible." And then Dr. Fothergill gives us his method of *rasping off the coating,* so to say, with "a compound calomel and colocynthe pill every second night, and a mixture of nitro-hydrochloric or phosphoric acid, with infusion of cinchona three times a day until the tongue clears." I would suggest that *nitro-glycerine* would act more speedily and reduce the suffering to a minimum! The point, however, to dwell upon,—and it is one worthy of the deepest consideration,—is that the state of the alimentary canal, so aptly described by the authority quoted, and which forbids the absorption of iron and oil, also prohibits the absorption of wholesome substances. Not only this; the secretion of the digestive fluids (even supposing for the moment that these fluids are present in normal amount and quality in the circulation, which is, of course, far from the truth in this as in most disorders) is in great degree prevented by this same physical obstruction, the "thick layer of dead epithelial cells;" and, moreover, the secretion of fecal matters by the glands of the colon is, in like manner and degree, prevented. (See chapter on "Constipation.")

What have we, then, in summing up, as the effect of this conservative effort of nature to "iron-sheathe and copper-fasten" this most abused alimentary tract, if I may thus characterize the coat which has resulted from the maltreatment of the digestive organs, and but for which the individual would, we may reasonably suppose, have died long ago from some plethoric disease? First: the digestive fluids, being scant and scantily secreted, it results that (2) only a small quantity at best, of the most wholesome food, can be by them digested, and (3) absorption from the small intestines is equally difficult, even supposing that the appropriate "small quantity" of food possible to be digested has not been exceeded, which, in ordinary practice, is anything but a supposable case. Excess is the invariable rule, and therefore (4) the undigested and fermenting food substances, excepting a portion which is absorbed in this poisonous condition, make their sluggish course along the intestines, collect in great masses in the lower bowel, and, finally, (a) either by aid of purgative medicines, or the ordinary stimulating drinks indulged in, (b) the irritating effects of these abnormal accumulations themselves, or (c) by means of injections, the lower bowel is more or less frequently emptied. These extraordinary evacuations are often described by the patient or friends as "exhausting." That such excreta is not composed of true fecal matters, we may reasonably conclude from the fact that (1) digestion and assimilation are but poorly performed, and but a very small proportion, therefore, of the quantity swallowed (often enough consumptives continue large eaters, gauged by any standard, and, relatively speaking, this is invariably the rule with them)—but a small proportion, I repeat, is absorbed into the circulation, and, therefore, undigested food must form the chief share of the so-called fecal matters, and (2) owing to the heavy fur-coat, lining the colon, the secretion of waste matters from the blood is, as just stated, well nigh prohibited.

Hence it results that under the ordinary treatment the consumptive patient is hurried out of the world by a relative, and, often enough, by an actual, exaggeration of the very practices which originated his disorder. Referring once more to Dr. Fothergill's, which is, to be sure, the regular drug plan: having scoured off the fur, so to say, with drastic purgatives, which have, possibly, cut a little too deep; or when, from whatever cause, instead of the furred coat, "the tongue is raw, bare, and denuded of epithelium, the patient should," he says, "take a mixture of *bismuth* with an *alkali* and use a milk diet. Seltzer water and milk will often agree when the milk alone is found to be too heavy and constipating." Here we have a case analogous to that of the robust gourmand whose dinner of a dozen courses is carried on and out by the aid of his "dinner pill," or the free use of filthy mineral waters: A cup or two of cow's milk (which, at best, is only a natural aliment for the calf, and which is too often drawn from a creature herself suffering from tuberculosis), is, to the depraved consumptive, even more "heavy and constipating" than the grossest diet indulged in ordinarily, to supposably healthy Christians, not to speak of such occasions as church festivals or society "breakfasts." One secret of the difficulty which besets the hygienist in his efforts to prevail upon a consumptive patient to persist in a course of "natural medication," after having once fairly entered upon it, lies in this: There is naturally a letting down, at first, from the stimulated condition, and this is often discouraging; the craving for the customary stimulants is almost as unappeasable as that of the rum-dyspeptic; and what makes the matter worse with the consumptive than with the drunkard, everybody who approaches the former seeks to tempt the appetite: or, in any event, the sight, smell, and hearing of the "good things" renders abstinence from such most difficult; and then, again, after leaving off many objectionable articles of food and drink, and having abstained from them for a few months, we will say, the transient resumption, always imminent, of the use of forbidden fruit operates with renewed force, and the patient finds himself, as he thinks, "gaining a little," and he is thus encouraged to fall back, more or less gradually, into all his old practices. Coffee, for example,—which originally proved constipating, after its first (laxative) effects ceased,—having been abstained from for some months, is now found to "agree" with and even "help" the patient, who, beginning with a single small cup at breakfast, works up finally to two at each meal; and, altogether, things go on swimmingly for a time. Again, after a period of abstinence from flesh-food, pastry, spices, etc.—to guard against which nature has put the fur-coat upon the intestines, or, perhaps, it should be said that the wear and tear occasioned by all unwholesome articles introduced into the stomach, have produced an effect somewhat analogous to the thickened cuticle resulting from the constant chafing of an ill-fitting shoe, for example,—as the intestinal tract begins to acquire something of its normal condition, there is a point when the resumption of a "generous" diet, in which the aforesaid substances figure largely, will seem to give the patient a fresh impulse healthward: they once more, perhaps, produce the laxative effects simulating that most desirable state of the bowels called "regular." And so on to the end of the chapter, the patient, friends, and perhaps the medical adviser, are misled as to the real state of affairs, until, finally, the end approaches, and the patient who was "improving so nicely" grows worse, and, after a period of intense suffering, which weans him from all desire to live, and reconciles his friends to the change, dies. "He caught cold, it settled on his lungs, and in his weak state"—etc., etc.

Speaking in round terms, the consumptive's digestive ability is about on a par, usually, indeed, inferior to his muscular powers; and it is as irrational to expect him to digest and assimilate several meals a day, as to expect him to saw several cords of wood in the same length of time. Both are alike impossible. The fact that the food disappears, or that there is a craving for it, even, or, again, that it "seems to agree with the stomach," does not change the case. A little food of the simplest sort may be assimilated, a little muscular exercise may be taken, and both prove curative. In common practice, however, the alimentary system is taxed to its own exhaustion and the impairment of the entire organism, while the voluntary muscular system deteriorates by reason of *non-use* as well as from the general lack of nutrition.

A very grave error, however, is sometimes made—of taking too much exercise; that is, of beginning the change too abruptly. Whatever the state of one's general health, he can only do with advantage *about* what he has *habitually done*. If he has all along lived a very active life and is in his usual health, he can take a good deal of exercise without harm, even with advantage; if, on the other hand, his life is sedentary, but little can be taken —beyond the current amount—without doing more harm than good. In either case, however, there may be a gradual increase of muscular exercise, and for many of the latter class this would prove life conserving, (if persisted in as a habit of life), but spasmodic efforts at building up a muscular system will always fail; nature does nothing in that fashion. The rule should be to exercise a little short of fatigue, and it should be increased little by little each day, "until the labor of working accommodates itself to easy habits." This rule would leave for some consumptive patients, at first, only the passive exercise of having their muscles pressed by their attendant's hand, or a gentle walk for a short distance, and so on.

"Combined with a hectic flush of the face, night-sweats, or general emaciation, shortness of breath leaves no doubt that the person thus affected is in the first stage of pulmonary consumption. If the patient were my son, I should remove the windows of his bedroom, and make him pass his days in the open air—as a cow-boy or berry-gatherer, if he could do no better. In case the disease had reached its *deliquium* period, the stage of violent bowel-complaints, dropsical swellings, and utter prostration,[23] it would be better to let the sufferer die in peace; but, as long as he were able to digest a frugal meal and walk two miles on level ground, I should begin the outdoor cure at any time of the year, and stake my own life on the result. I should provide him with clothing enough to defy the vicissitudes of the seasons, and keep him outdoors in all kinds of weather—walking, riding, or sitting; he would be safe: the fresh air would prevent the *progress* of the disease. But *improve* he could not without exercise. Increased exercise is the price of increased vigor. Running and walking steel the leg-sinews. In order to strengthen his wrist-joints a man must handle heavy weights. Almost any bodily exercise—but especially swinging, wood-chopping, carrying weights, and walking up-hill—increases the action of the lungs, and thus gradually their functional vigor. Gymnastics that expand the chest facilitate the action of the respiratory organs, and have the collateral advantage of strengthening the sinews, and invigorating the system in general, by accelerating every function of the vital process. The exponents of the movement-cure give a long list of athletic evolutions, warranted to widen out the chest as infallibly as French-horn practice expands the cheeks. But the trouble with such machine-exercises is that they are almost sure to be discontinued as soon as they have relieved a momentary distress, and, as Dr.

Pitcher remarks in his 'Memoirs of the Osage Indians,' the symptoms of consumption (caused by smoking and confinement in winter quarters) disappear during their annual buffalo-hunt, but reappear upon their return to the indolent life of the wigwam. The problem is to make outdoor exercise pleasant enough to be permanently preferable to the *far niente* whose sweets seem especially tempting to consumptives. This purpose accomplished, the steady progress of convalescence is generally insured, for the differences of climate, latitude, and altitude, of age and previous habits, almost disappear before the advantages of an habitual outdoor life over the healthiest indoor occupations."—("Physical Education.")

[23] The fasting consumptive referred to on page 62 had already approached this condition.—AUTHOR.

I would not be understood, by any means, as advising every consumptive patient, or every one who supposes himself to be suffering from this disease, to immediately and without advice stop eating; but this much I do say: in all cases of progressive emaciation, that is to say, where the organs of digestion and assimilation have become so impaired that the body is not nourished, but is steadily declining, the attending physician should *consider* the question of temporary rest for the alimentary organs, so far as the ingestion of food is concerned. The presence even of a craving appetite should be treated as a morbid symptom, and should weigh in favor of abstinence. It should also be borne in mind that the earlier this remedy is applied the smaller will be the "dose" indicated, and the more speedy and complete the relief. Had Mr. Connolly, for example—whose cure by fasting I have already alluded to—at any time during his first few months of "pressure at the lungs, with cough and expectoration," fasted for a week or ten days,[24] perhaps, under the care of a physician sufficiently intelligent to judge of his needs in this direction, and had he thereafter lived on the plain diet which he now finds so complete, he would in all probability have escaped the illness which followed, and would have enjoyed uninterrupted health to the present day. Again, if he had changed his manner of living five years earlier—from three "mixed" meals[25] of stimulating food, as flesh and the irritating condiments invariably associated with animal food; pastry, white flour, and stimulating drinks, as tea and coffee—to two meals composed of the cereals, vegetables and fruits, prepared in the simplest and plainest manner, there would have been no call for a fast. I have the means of knowing of over five thousand families in this country alone who have made this change for preventive and curative purposes, and with the happiest results. I would say that any person who finds his appetite failing or fitful—sometimes poor, sometimes craving—and who has reason to fear the decline of his nutritive powers, will do well to make a radical change in his habits of living; and the sooner the better. The most pernicious custom of which I have any knowledge, yet one almost universal in the care of the sick, is that of "tempting the appetite," concocting fancy or especially toothsome dishes, when nature is saying in the plainest manner that feeding has already been overdone. Such preparations are a severe tax upon even robust persons—they are fatal to consumptives. It is infinitely worse than bribing an exhausted laborer, who can scarcely move a muscle, to rouse himself to fresh tasks. He will do more and better work by reason of present and absolute rest; and the same is true of the sick stomach: there will be a relish for the coarsest article of diet—aye, it will be delicious—and digestion will wait on appetite, when the nutritive organs shall have been restored by sufficient rest. The experiments of Tanner at New York, Griscomb at Chicago, and now of Terrence Connolly (the consumptive faster) at Newton, N. J., have, I believe, demonstrated the fact that, in health or in sickness, in all cases of abstinence from all food, saving only water and pure air, of whatever disease the subject may die, it will not be for want of food, *so long as there remains any considerable amount of flesh*[26] *on his bones*. By the light of these experiences we shall do well, too, to study more closely the functions of the lymphatic system: human flesh, by absorption, constitutes a most appropriate diet in certain conditions of disease (see article on rheumatism). The absorption and excretion of diseased tissues is, under some circumstances, the only work that nature can with safety undertake, and in these cases no building up can be accomplished until a solid foundation is reached and the *debris* removed; and *not then unless, while this good work is going on, the nutritive organs are given an opportunity to virtually renew themselves.*

[24] It is evident that such a fast, *then*, would have proved, so far as the danger of starvation is concerned, a mere bagatelle, since three years later, as we have seen,—years of decline and emaciation,—he endured, and, with advantage, a fast of over six weeks.

[25] A return to his old diet now would probably make short work of this subject, and should I hear of his early death, my first inquiry would relate to this point.

[26] The amount "consumed" in the case of Mr. Connolly from day to day, was very slight indeed, scarcely more than before he left off eating; that is, it was observed that his emaciation was no more rapid during the fast than immediately prior thereto; before the fast his food was not being digested nor assimilated, and he was taking purgatives continually for torpid bowels.

Dr. Tanner, in his forty days' fast, lost about fifty pounds in weight. Mr. Griscomb lost a little more than that in his fast of forty-five days; and although moving about, taking more exercise every day than many sedentary people, and attending to a large correspondence, etc., was still able to say to the audience assembled to see him break his fast: "Ladies and gentlemen, you see now a man who has swallowed no food, except water, for forty-five days, and yet I can assure you that I am neither faint nor hungry; but I shall soon convince you that I have an excellent appetite," and, so saying, he proceeded to partake of a very moderate dinner, and in moderate fashion. It is commonly supposed that these are uncommon men: they are uncommon only in possessing a knowledge as to the power of the living organism to withstand abstinence from food, and in having the courage of their opinions. And yet, when discussing the advantages of the two-meal system, uninformed people talk about "getting faint if they go so long" without nourishment! They speak from the three-meal-fish-flesh-fowl and pickle stand-point; accustomed to applying a hot poultice to a gnawing, sick stomach every few hours, they do get faint if the time runs over a single hour.

These various fasts, with the lessons to be drawn from them, must prove, finally, of inestimable value to science in the treatment of disease, where it may be desirable to rest all the viscera, or any portion thereof, concerned in digestion,[27] or to "close the bowels" for certain surgical operations, without resorting to injurious medication, and also—a very important consideration—in cases of enforced abstinence, as in time of famine or shipwreck, to prevent death from fright and discouragement, which have heretofore killed scores where actual starvation has one.

[27] An eminent Maine statesman has recently died, who might have recovered and lived for years, but for the mistaken theory that food is a daily need under all circumstances: To constantly feed an irritated stomach is like kicking a man when he is down. And yet this is being done with fatal effect constantly all over the world. In certain cases, and especially with aged patients, this system is as surely fatal as strychnine, if less speedy. There are many besides myself who believe that President Garfield died from fatty degeneration, chronic dyspepsia, and constant feeding during his illness, rather than from the effects of the bullet. True enough, he might have lived on for years in his disordered physical condition but for the wound; still, on the other hand, it is equally probable that he might have lived, and that his sickness would have restored him to health even, but for the constant tampering with his stomach, which needed rest as much as the great and good man himself. No rest for the stomach, no rest for the man, is an axiom which I would submit to my brother practitioners, as one worthy of all acceptation. It is being constantly proved right before their own eyes, and yet very few have learned the lesson it teaches.

As illustrating the influence of an out-door life, with partial or transient fasting, I will cite

THE CASE OF MR. VICKERS.

Joseph Vickers, born and raised in England, but now of Biddeford, Me., whose home is near my own, and the man himself well known to me, was very "low with consumption" at one time, when in his twenty-second year. His disease was attributed, and without doubt justly, to a severe chill resulting from wading the river on one of his hunting bouts, and being compelled to dry his clothes on his back—a feat he had previously performed repeatedly, except that on this occasion, being very much fatigued, and night coming on, instead of continuing vigorous exercise while his clothes were drying, he "went into camp" and "shivered throughout the night in his soaked garments." Declining very rapidly, with every symptom of pulmonary consumption, his case was considered hopeless by his friends. Medicine seeming to him useless, he gave up taking it, and his physician consequently gave him no encouragement or hope of recovery. His digestion was very imperfect—as he put it, "Nothing I ate seemed to do me any good"—and to the disgust of his parents and friends he often refused to eat anything for an entire day. Able to be up and dressed a good portion of the time, he would spend as much of the day outdoors as possible, and at night "never slept without a window open in the bedroom." Gaining a little strength, and being "badgered," as he says, "all the time, when at home, about eating," and being very fond of hunting, and not sleeping well, he would rise very early, take his gun and, as he expressed it, would "crawl off to the woods," and sit or lie down until rested, and then "travel a bit and rest again," and so spend the entire day, taking no lunch, and eating nothing, drinking from a brook or a spring when thirsty, returning at night, often as late as seven or eight o'clock, when he would eat a little coarse food after resting, and then go to bed. "A couple of weeks" of this sort of life sufficed to bring him home at night with an "appetite for a side of sole-leather," and he would eat a hearty supper—always of the plainest food—and soon go to bed. From this point his recovery was as rapid as his decline had been. His diet has always been of the plainest sort, mostly vegetable (a large proportion of coarse bread and fruit),—"My drink is always cold water, and I let the rest of the family eat all the fancy stuff," he remarked. Mr. Vickers,—who is a devout Christian man, and his story corroborated in every feature by others as reliable,—is now sixty-six years old, though he appears like a robust, well-preserved man of fifty.

Excepting under very aggravated conditions, as for example, the case of Mr. Vickers, given above, rarely does any creature ever *begin* to have consumption with a sound stomach, liver, and intestines. Nor can the digestive organs become diseased, ordinarily, so long as the diet and general regimen are even approximately correct. If we thought more of what would "tickle" the stomach and intestines than the palate, simply, we would banish most of our disorders; pure air, active exercise, a *clear conscience*, and the cultivation of a spirit of cheerfulness, kindliness, and contentment, would send the balance a-flying. Upon the importance of cheerfulness, a recent writer, a physician with a large practice, and a man of keen perceptions, says: "One of the most important directions of all is personal and subjective. Cultivate with the utmost force possible the habit of cheerfulness. No words can put this out with the strength and weight which I should be glad to give to it. Its value is utterly beyond estimation. The difference between meeting the common, or uncommon, trials of life with cheerfulness or with despondency, and perhaps complaint and grumbling, is often just the difference between life and death."

The appetite for "sweets"—candy, syrup, sugar, and fancy dishes deluged with sweet sauces—encouraged to an abnormal degree from infancy, and the gratification of this appetite throughout life are prolific aids in establishing the phthisical diathesis. There is a natural appetite for *sweet fruits* and this demand may be safely met by such forms of food, but never by the unbalancing artificial sweets, or *proximate principles* of food, as cane or beet sugar and the "bon-bons" formed from them.

Victor Hugo,—that grand man who gave us "*Les Miserables*,"—in the first volume of the series, puts this bit of physiological wisdom into the mouth of the witty libertine, Tholomyés, who uses it, to be sure, in a double sense, which I need not here explain: "Now, listen attentively!" says this oracle of the "four." "Sugar is a salt. Every salt is desiccating. Sugar is the most desiccating of all salts. It sucks up the liquids from the blood through the veins; thence comes the coagulation, then the solidification of the blood; thence the tubercles in the lungs; thence death. And this is why diabetes borders on consumption." I commend the above thought to consumptives, and to the parents of fat children—the consumptives of the future. Every grain of artificial sugar swallowed, constitutes a tax upon the system—upon the lungs and kidneys, more particularly—a tax upon the individual's vitality.

Among the prolific causes of consumption in after life, is that of the involuntary cramming and fattening of infancy, followed up during childhood and youth by a somewhat less excessive gluttony, which is taught inferentially by the conversation and example of the elders, as by constantly dwelling upon the delights of the palate, arranging entertainments which are feasts of the body, rather than of the mind, in advance of which all classes discuss with excess of interest the palatal pleasures of the coming "good time," and at which all unite, if not in gorging themselves, at least in feeding themselves for pleasure to the disregard of the true requirements of their bodies for nutriment.

As a result of all this, sedentary persons become, like stall-fed oxen, degenerated with fat; and this, as just remarked about children, is a predisposing cause of consumption. A very large proportion of consumptives, most of them, in fact, are first thus diseased; and when any person is round and plump, or even fairly covered, so to say, and is yet lacking in muscular power—"easily tired"—it is *prima facie* evidence that the muscular system is degenerated in the manner described; and if the muscles, then the vital organs within, also. Thus we observe that grossness is by no means essential to fatty degeneration, although all obese persons are, of course, thus affected.

The salary of a fireman ("coal heaver") depends upon his intelligence in the matter of fuelling up his engine with a view to its "health," power and longevity; that of the cook or caterer, upon his ingenuity in devising means to accomplish the reverse of all this in the case of the human engine placed at his mercy.

"A well-spread board" should be described as one at which the youngest child (whose teeth are cut) may exercise his will without let or hindrance until, at the first indication of dallying, or "loafing," over his food, it is evident that he has had enough; and at which the consumptive may eat without being tempted to overindulge, but, paying heed to the first intimation of satiety, rise from the table with the assurance of having performed an agreeable duty, in that he has eaten in quantity and quality, what he can digest and assimilate. The consumptive starves, not for want of food, but for want of digestion and assimilation. It is impossible to emphasize this fact too strongly.

The *Scientific American* of June 3, 1882, in an article entitled "Tubercle Parasite,"[28] considering Dr. Koch's theory, says: "According to Dr. Salisbury, this disease (consumption) is one arising from 'continued unhealthy alimentation, and must be treated by removing the cause. This cause is fermenting food and the products of this fermentation, viz.: alcoholic yeast and alcohol, vinegar yeast and acetic acid, carbonic acid gas, embolism, and interference with nutrition. Consumption of the bowels can be produced at any time in the human subject in from fifteen to thirty days, and consumption of the lungs inside of ninety days, by special, exclusive, and continued feeding upon the diet that produces them—that is, food containing starch and sugar in alcoholic and acetic acid fermentation.'" Dr. Salisbury had found this embryonic form of the vinegar yeast in the blood, sputa, and excretions of persons suffering with consumption. In the blood the plant forms masses by itself, grows inside the white corpuscles, causes the fibrin filaments of the blood to be larger in size and stronger, the red corpuscles to be ropy, sticky, adhesive, making small clots or "thrombi," which become "emboli" or plugs, and block up the capillaries and blood-vessels. The growth of the vinegar yeast in its embryonal stage, combined with the mechanical interference with nutrition, causes abnormal growths in the substance of organs, called tubercle; and the concurrent inflammatory results, in addition to the chemical action of the vinegar or acetic acid, causes the death and breaking down of the organs invaded—the lungs, for example. That this is not opinion only is shown by the fact that over 246 swine were, at his instance, destroyed by feeding on farinaceous food in a state of alcoholic and vinegar fermentation, the vinegar yeast traced in the blood, found in the excretions, and 104 of the dead swine were subjected to *post-mortem* examinations and their lungs found broken down and diseased as in ordinary consumption. The same experiment was tried on a number of men, "all healthy, and with no vegetations in the blood. They were given plenty of exercise in the open air," but within three months these men had consumption of the lungs. "Certainly," says the *Scientific American*, "we think the evidence submitted shows that Dr. Salisbury has come nearer to the real intimate nature of consumption than Dr. Koch or any one we know. There is a simplicity, directness, breadth, and positiveness rarely seen in the treatment of a medical subject. Indeed, it is doubtful if there have been experiments so conclusive and extensive before or since." It must be evident to even the crudest thinker that this fermenting process must ultimately produce the same effects when *begun in the stomach*, and described as indigestion; and no more efficient means of initiating this process can be imagined than that of swallowing indigestible substances—the most wholesome food-substances may be prepared in such a manner as to render them indigestible—or eating in excess of the needs of the organism, and therefore of the capacity for digestion. Thousands upon thousands of so-called healthy people are in this way approaching the point of decline, more or less slowly, but surely, utterly unconscious of their danger, simply because in their ignorance they can not recognize the premonitory symptoms, of which chronic constipation, for example, is one, and a very grave one. (See article on this subject.)

[28] Microscopic examination reveals the presence of a multiplicity of fatty crystals throughout the substance of the lungs of persons who have died of consumption. At a recent meeting of the New Orleans Pathological Society, its President, Dr. H. D. Schmidt, whose researches have been extended and minute, made an important microscopical demonstration to disprove Prof. Koch's so-called discovery as to the bacilli of tuberculosis. Prof. Schmidt claimed to demonstrate that the so-called bacilli, thought by Dr. Koch to be the cause of consumption, were simply fatty crystals. Connecting with this the fact that Prof. Koch really found certain minute living organisms which he propagated artificially for several generations, it becomes evident to my mind (1) that the "bacillus" is simply a natural scavenger enveloped in the diseased tissue—the fatty crystal, or the tubercle—and (2) that its office is really, under the circumstances, conservative to life. Nor is this conclusion disproved by the alleged fact that the inoculation with the bacilli, of *supposably* healthy animals, produced the disorder: In the first place, the little domestic pets, such as were thus operated upon, are always, owing to their artificial surroundings, predisposed to the disease in question, frequently falling victims to it without the aid of inoculation, and (3) this being the case, their inoculation with a liberal reinforcement of greedy vermin,—or, supposing that, as yet, none were generated, their premature introduction,—would naturally tend to a speedy and fatal termination. It makes no difference to a dead man whether his lungs were devoured by bacilli, or simply broken down from fatty degeneration; but to the living, it is a matter of the utmost importance to learn the true condition of things in the premises. The idea of being eaten alive by myriads of little vermin from which there is supposably no escape, is enough to strike terror to the mind of a patient; but let him know that his disease is of such a nature that (with the *aid* of the bacilli, perhaps,) a radical change in his manner of living affords great assurance for the hope of its entire eradication, and he has at once an all-sufficient motive for reform.

Dr. J. Milner Fothergill, in a letter to the *Philadelphia Medical Times*, referring to Koch's theory of the origin of tuberculosis, remarks, half jocosely: "Talk of the bitterness of death! It is nothing to the shadowy danger which overhangs us of a tubercle-bacillus getting into one's pulmonary alveoli in an unguarded moment, and when one's 'resistive power' happens to be impaired. Shadowy in the sense of invisible, not unreal! Is this what is meant by 'the doom of a great city'? Is the bacillus a relative of the poison-germ which slew Sennacherib's host in a night? We do not yet know the little creature intimately enough to say. But, really, the horrors which the mind conjures up of the dangers of the bacillus in the future are demoralizing. Suppose, now, that some change of the human constitution should favor the bacillus, just as the potato-field did the Colorado beetle, who had been happily quiet in his dietary of the leaves of the deadly nightshade, but who went on the war-path when the leaves of the other members of the Solanaceæ came within his reach. The imagination fails to conceive what may be the fate of man,—to be slain by a foe more remorseless than any of the plagues of Egypt. Suppose, now, that the bacillus took such a new departure, and got ahead of our 'resistive power.' Why, man would be swept off the face of the earth! What an ignominious end, too! Man, in the plenitude of his power over the forces of nature, slain by an insignificant little bacillus!"

After all, excess in diet is, usually, only another term for lack of fresh air and exercise, without which no one can become, or continue, robust. While it is true that to command health and muscular vigor one must be well fed, still no amount of food alone can make the right arm like that of a blacksmith. But we can make the muscles grow on ample exercise and—food enough; always, however, considering a constant supply of oxygen as an essential element in the ration. The muscular system wastes—with many is never even tolerably developed—the powers wane, because of sedentary habits. "Inaction contravenes the supreme design of the human constitution, and is therefore adverse to its health."—HUXLEY. The lungs begin to take on disease, often, because the individual does nothing to make him *breathe deep*; exercise is not frequent and vigorous[29] enough to cause frequent deep inspirations; the remote air-cells are in many instances seldom, and with corset-wearers *never*, inflated, and, consequently, the tendency is to grow together, so to say, or, rather, to fester and slough off, as useless appendages. To form the habit of taking long breaths in the open air, occasionally, throughout the day, would do much to maintain the integrity of lung-tissue, aerate the blood and prevent or cure consumption; but, after all, Nature designs that creatures who inhabit this earth shall be "fit" for something besides drawing their own breath.[30] To be "fit to survive" one must be of use in the world; hence there must be employment that taxes the mental, moral, and physical forces sufficiently to stimulate their growth and development. This, and nothing short of this, is health, in the complete sense of the term. *Robust health*, if one would secure it, demands that one should be much in the open air and exposed, often, to a low temperature while taking a great deal of vigorous exercise. To be *long-lived*, on the other hand, requires rather that the diet be restricted to correspond with abstinence from labor and cold, some degree of exercise in the open air, however, being essential. The robust often wear out faster than the brain workers, whose lives are rather on the quiet order. Worry kills ten where work kills one.

[29] In a badly vitiated atmosphere *inaction* is the only palliative; muscular exercise causes a demand for an increased supply of oxygen, and increases the amount of carbonic acid to be eliminated, neither of which conditions can be met except by means of pure air.

[30] See note 1 in Appendix, p. 275.

The best illustration of the natural means of preventing, or curing, consumption—in fact, of promoting and maintaining health, under any circumstances—I have ever seen, is given in the following true story of

HOW A YOUNG GIRL CURED HERSELF.

"Then you are surprised to learn that I came within six weeks of dying of consumption, thirty years ago, are you, doctor?" The questioner was a bright, healthy little woman of fifty who, in the course of a consultation about a consumptive niece, had expressed herself as having little hope of her recovery, "because she wouldn't do as I did when I had the disease—and she isn't nearly as sick as I was." Straight as an arrow, active and merry, looking more like forty than fifty, Mrs. E. was the last person that any one would select as belonging to a "consumptive family," or of having suffered with the disease, in her own person, and yet her mother died of it when this daughter was about 19, and the latter's decline was attributed to inherited tendency and long confinement in the sick-room, during the last year of her mother's life. "Yes, I have told Lettie how I cured myself after the doctors gave me up, but she will not undertake it—not now, at least—perhaps she may when she gets where I was. Do you want me to give you my recipe for the cure of consumption, Doctor? Tell you the whole story? Well, the way is simple, and the story a short one, and if it will help any one I shall be very glad. I needn't tell you all about mother's case—hers was the old-fashioned consumption; she was sick a good many years, but the last year she was almost helpless and would have no one but me to take care of her. Well, I bore up until she died, and then I gave out; I could not go to the grave—I was in bed during the funeral. I had not realized—none of the family had—how poorly I had become; but now it was plain enough. I kept my bed most of the time—could not get rested. I had been sick several weeks when my brother was brought home ill, was taken with typhoid fever, and there was no one to nurse him. I roused myself up and declared that I was able to do it; and I carried the point, in spite of all father could say. Well, he was sick nine weeks, but I gave up before he recovered. I carried him through the worst of it, however, before I took my bed; and then I was very sick indeed. For a while they thought I could live but a few weeks, but I rallied and got more comfortable. I raised a great deal, and for several months remained about the same, apparently; but the autumn came, and when we began to shut the house up I seemed to grow worse; my cough was still very bad, but I couldn't 'raise' much, and I suffered terribly for breath. The doctor who had been attending me—the one who had tended mother—at last said he could do no more for me, and for some months we had no physician, and then father called a new one—a young doctor who was fitting himself for practice in our village. He came to see me, examined my lungs, and I fainted away in the effort. He went out—leaving no medicine—and had a talk with father. He said that he did not care to take the case; that there was no hope for me; my lungs were badly ulcerated, and I had but few weeks to live. 'She can't live over six weeks,[31] Mr. B., and she may die any day. I am young, just commencing practice, and it will injure me to have her die on my hands; and I can not help her.' 'At least,' said father, 'give her something to relieve her suffering.' They did not know that I could hear them; but spring-time had come again, the day was quite warm, and I had asked to have the window raised at the head of my bed, and so it happened that I could hear all they said. I heard the doctor returning, and I resolved not to take any of his soothing drops; I had taken all I meant to. 'Well,' said I, 'what have you come back for, doctor?' 'Your father wished me to prescribe for you,' said he. 'Never mind,' I said, firmly, 'I shall take nothing more. You say I have six weeks to live: I will spend them in getting rid of the medicines I have taken the past year,' and he went away. Soon father came in, seeming much disappointed and grieved, and in answer to his questioning, I told him why I had determined to take no more medicine, and what I had resolved to do; and now I will tell you what I did, and how I came to do it. I had read in an old English almanac—not a medical one, like the ones strewn about everywhere now, but there was a good deal of useful information in it—a 'Sure Cure for Consumption,' and it was so different from what I had been doing, and appealed so strongly to my judgment, that I had been thinking that if I could only make a start there might be a chance for me; but the effort required was so great that I doubt if I should have had courage enough to undertake it but for my resentment, upon overhearing that conversation—to think that the doctors had given me nothing but medicine, and that I had been eating in such a way—without any appetite, except for some of the 'rich' things they were always making because I couldn't relish anything else. The recipe explained that the disease was caused by lack of fresh air, outdoor exercise, and appropriate food; but I will only tell you what I did, and you will understand all about the reasons for it. First, I told father and the rest of the family that as I had but six weeks to live, they must let me have my own way in everything, and must do as I said. I could not move from the bed alone, but I had them carry me on a comforter out on the lawn and lay me down there. 'How was *I* to take exercise—when I could scarcely turn myself in bed?' was the question. Well, I did turn myself on one side, and, with a stick, begun to dig a little in the ground. It looked then as though I should not do much damage to the nice sod father had taken so much pains to make; but I dug a little hole as large as my fist, and then rested. After a while I turned over on the other side and dug another little hole, filled it up, and rested again. It seemed good to rest and I felt a little better; for the outdoor air, and the exertion I had put forth, 'loosened' my cough a little, and I begun to 'raise.' At night they carried me back to bed. My bed-room windows had been wide open all day, and I wouldn't have them shut now; but in answer to their fears about the night air and catching cold, I said, 'Give me clothes enough, and I will risk the night air—I'm going to breathe pure air the next six weeks—if I live so long.' They all felt terribly—they thought I was shortening my life, even then—but they yielded, finally, in everything, even to not asking me 'if I couldn't eat a little of this, or that, if they would make it for me?' I had replied: 'No, when I feel like eating a piece of Graham bread or a potato, without butter or salt, I will eat something—not before.' This had occurred in the morning, and that very night I asked for a slice of bread and ate a little bit—as big as my two fingers, perhaps. I had them put a teaspoonful of cayenne pepper[32] in a dish and turn warm water on it—a quart—and let it stand overnight, and in the morning was sponged all over in that water—the dregs turned off. I had them bathe an arm and then dry it with a coarse towel, and rub me with it as hard as I could bear (not very hard, to be sure), then a leg, and so on.[33] It seemed to give the dead skin a little life; then they carried me out to my 'work' again! I felt like resting after the bath, but after a while I turned over and dug a larger hole than on the day before, filled it—partly with what I raised from my lungs, and such stuff as it was! I could take longer breaths, too; and after digging a minute or so I would *have* to stop and take a long breath, and then go on again.[34] I was thirsty a good deal, and would drink water—all I wanted. I ate a piece of stale coarse bread and some fruit that morning after I was rested from my first digging, and then I kept on resting for some hours, after which I dug a little more. In the middle of the day, when the sun came down too hot, I had an old umbrella put over me and fastened. At night a little bit of bread and a small potato: I ate as much as I could relish, but not a mouthful more. In this way I kept on, day after day, and they began to see that I was gaining. Father, who could not believe the gain was real, but rather the temporary effect of my will, yet joked me about ruining the lawn: 'I shall have to turf it all over again, Lucia,' said he, even before I could dig a hole large enough in a day to bury a cat in, and he tried to laugh at his little joke. I remember that I did laugh, and came near strangling in a coughing fit in consequence, but that was a help; what I *needed* was to cough and raise the stuff up—those old ulcers that the doctor said my lungs were covered with—and I found fresh air, flavored with a little exercise, a better 'expectorant,' as you doctors say, than those I had been taking. I began to feel hopeful—the novelty of the idea—digging for my life! I took a desperate view of it—six weeks to live—'I'll die fighting,' I said to myself. It seemed almost droll—droll enough, at any rate, to interest my mind, and I would say funny things to the others to make them laugh, and this seemed to make them try to be cheerful and to cheer me on. The third day, I remember that I ate the same kind of a breakfast—just a little—and at night asked them to boil a beet! I would have only one vegetable at a time, lest I might be tempted to overeat and lose my appetite, and so spoil everything.[35] I was impressed with the idea of 'earning my living' at outdoor work—'by the sweat of my brow'—and not to eat more than I earned by the exercise. I had renounced my coffee and tea; I ate no grease of any kind, nor meat—bread, fruit, and vegetables only—no salt or spices, pastry, pie, puddings, nor cake, nor 'sweets' of any sort, except the natural, *whole* sweet furnished by nature, in the form of vegetables and sweet fruits. The prescription said that some people ate too much soft food,—bread and milk, puddings, and the like,—and that while such dishes were better than many others in common use, still they were not the best, especially for sick people with weak stomachs, but that dry (farinaceous) food was every way better; and so I ate bread, or unleavened biscuit, which, after a little practice, the girl could make very nice,—just the meal and water well mixed and moulded stiff and baked in a hot oven,—and I ate them very slowly, chewing each mouthful thoroughly. You can tell, perhaps, doctor, just why this should make a difference:[36] I only know that it seemed to agree with my stomach better. They bathed me every morning in the same way, only after a while they did not have to work so slowly and cautiously. I could exercise more and more, from day to day, and with less and less fatigue, and I laughed to myself that father's joke would prove something more than a joke; I was bound to undo all his nice work; and I knew he wouldn't care, so that I could get well. After a while I could raise myself up and sit erect, and dig a little, first on one side and then on the other; and by the time my 'six weeks' were up—and I told father so one day—I could dig a pretty good grave for myself, if they wanted to bury me; only, it wouldn't be quite deep enough to hold me down—for I had actually raised myself to my feet, stood alone, and walked a few steps without help. On the eighth week I could walk about—would walk off a dozen steps, come back, sit down—perhaps lie down. The more I did, the more I could do—always taking care not to exhaust myself—and the more I could eat; but I took even more care not to overeat than not to overwork: I found that the real thing was to eat little enough—not to see how much I could eat—so that I could increase the amount regularly, rather than to lose my appetite and eat nothing some days, or eat without an appetite, and next day eat enormously, perhaps, as mother used to; I wouldn't have them 'fix up' anything—I was afraid of being put back. I ate but twice a day, and sometimes my breakfast was nothing but fruit—two or three oranges or as many apples, or a huge slice of watermelon—this was food and drink, both. I wore the least possible weight of clothing—often removing my stockings as well as shoes, and going barefooted and bare-armed when the weather was very warm. I had lost all fear of taking cold, though I kept comfortable always—throwing off clothing when too warm, and putting it on, as any great change in the temperature made it necessary, but to the extent of my increasing strength I endeavored to keep warm by exerting my muscles. One day, after some months of self-treatment, and when it had become evident that I was really convalescent, I asked brother to call Dr. Osgood (the young doctor who refused to take my case). 'Why, sis,' said he, 'you are not in earnest?' 'Yes, I am,' said I, 'I want to tell him how to cure consumption! You tell him I want to see him, but don't say what for.' He had been away somewhere, and had forgotten all about me, of course, but when brother spoke to him about me, he was astonished to find that I was alive. 'It was amazing' he said. 'Yes, if there is any chance of saving(!) her I will call'—and he came. He expressed his pleasure at finding me so well, and I suppose he thought I had come to a point where I felt the need of his advice and a 'tonic,' perhaps; but I just made him listen to the story of my self-cure, and asked him if he couldn't advise others to do the same way, and so do his patients more good. He was inclined to be vexed, at first, but finally he laughed and said: 'Really, Miss B———, I have come here at your request, and you have prescribed for me, instead of I for you, and I thank you for it—will pay you for it, if you will name the price—but I could not practice in that way. Why, how many consumptives would act upon my advice, if it was of that character? How many, indeed, would have the second visit from me, or recommend me to others? They would even denounce me to their friends—to every one they saw, and I would have to go to digging in the ground myself, or leave for other parts. No, Miss B

———, you learned the true secret, and you were "fit" to "survive" because you worked out your own salvation: you have taught me something—a valuable lesson, I may say, and one that I shall profit by as I have an opportunity; but we could never set up such a reform—one doctor, nor two, nor three, alone—the time is not ripe for it, physicians are not ripe for it, and it can only come, if it is ever to come, by just such independent action as your case represents.' And so he went away, and I continued my 'treatment.' The next summer I had a little flower garden of my own, watered and tended it, and, a little later, helped about the kitchen-garden, besides taking care of my own room; and so I went on, gaining steadily, until, within two years, I was well—better than I had known myself since my romping days, and I have scarcely had a real sick day since—never a serious illness from that day to this, nearly thirty years." "How do I keep well?" you ask. "Why, by pursuing the same principle that cured me—the same, in fact, that would have prevented my decline, in the first place. I never breathe 'indoor' air, winter nor summer, day nor night; I eat only the simplest food, and in moderation—yet I will, sometimes, eat a little more than I need—some meals or some days—and will have a little headache, or, perhaps, an old tooth will ache, or there may be a little disturbance in the stomach; but whatever it is, I eat more moderately—sometimes go without a meal; and if anything more serious than I have named presents itself— lack of appetite, or a bad feeling at the stomach, or a bad headache—I go all day without eating, and keep about my work, as usual, or take a walk outdoors, and this plan always works a cure. You see, I *dress* right—loose garments, no corsets, no heavy skirts hanging to my waist or hips, no smothering flannels, except the lightest, and those only in the coldest weather; I keep busy about something most of the time; take a good deal of exercise; go out when I can, and bring outdoors in when I can't go out—by having every part of my house well ventilated and as light and 'sunshiny' as need be (you see, doctor, I am not whimsically afraid of flies nor of fading the carpet); I think of my escape, of my good health, and this makes me cheerful. I feel sure of not getting sick—I have no anxiety on that score,— and I try to do what good I can, in my small way, and all this is as it should be—it is 'healthy,' and, all things being so, there is only one other chance to err, and that is in eating, and so when anything troubles me, I know what it is. So many people go wrong in all these things—dress bad, breathe bad air, feel languid in consequence and lie about doing nothing, indoors; eat worse food than I do, and eat more and oftener—no wonder they are always ailing, nor that so many die. But, Doctor, this will not cure my niece—our talking—and I don't suppose I have taught you anything, as I did the young doctor, so many years ago; but if, as you say, you can tell the story for the benefit of others, I shall be very glad indeed to see it in print. You will send me a copy of the paper, won't you? 'A dozen copies?' Well, all the better, I will send them to my friends; they will wonder how the 'old story' got into the papers." And that is the way this history of a "Natural Cure" came to be printed.

[31] It is, of course, idle to speculate as to whether Miss B. was within six weeks, or six months, of a fatal termination of her disease under the usual treatment. Her physician expressed his honest opinion, certainly; though had he been catechised closely, he would doubtless have modified it somewhat, as, by saying that while she was liable to be taken off at any time, still, she might linger along several months, or until severe cold weather in winter, the season usually so fatal to this class of patients,—not because it is impossible, or even difficult, to keep the sick-room at any desired temperature, but because this end is sought to be accomplished, largely, by shutting out "the breath of life," and by retaining the vitiated air, to breathe which would "chill" the healthiest subject. "To retain foul air for the sake of its warmth is expensive economy."

[32] It was, in the author's opinion, the *bath* rather than the *pepper* which proved so beneficial.

[33] In practice, it will often prove that quick sponging, all over, and brisk drying, followed, perhaps, by thorough hand-rubbing, will be more useful than the "piece-meal" bath: with water at a comfortable temperature, and the work quickly and skillfully performed, while it might seem likely to occasion a severe shock to the patient, still, it is but one "shock" instead of many, and is really far less trying, with many patients, than the more prolonged process with its oft-repeated local shocks. If rightly managed, the reaction from the full bath makes it altogether the most agreeable. It is of vital importance, to secure this warm "reaction," and if, in any instance, there is failure in this direction, the instant application of warming appliances—hot-water bottles to feet, warm flannel wraps, extra blankets, etc.—is imperatively demanded. Baths which are succeeded by chilliness are depleting, and if of common occurrence are destructive to life; far better not bathe at all.

[34] See note 6 in Appendix, p. 284.

[35] One element which aided immensely in this remarkable cure, was the absence of great variety in the food. Indigestion is *the* enemy to be overcome; and he must be "killed dead." *Variety* is this enemy's right-hand man—encouraging excess and the indulgence in questionable articles; and, above all, prohibiting the *adaptation* of the digestive organs to any class of all the ailments thrust upon them. (See foot-note, p. 213.)

[36] The "difference" is in the digestibility, and in guarding against excess: Overeating is, of itself, a positive guarantee of indigestion.[A] The advantages of the hard bread and "dry diet" are manifold: (1) thorough mastication—calling the muscles of the mouth into action, and while this tends to make the cheeks plump and full, the exercise affects the various glands, and aids in the secretion of the salivary fluids essential for the digestion of starch;[B] (2) it causes one to eat slowly, so that each mouthful entering the stomach; is not only thoroughly insalivated and thus prepared for stomach-digestion, but can be thoroughly manipulated in the stomach and impregnated completely with the gastric juice: this must be deemed a very important feature, when we reflect that in very depraved states the digestive fluids are not as abundant nor as readily secreted as in health. (3) Chewing strengthens the gums and the teeth,—tends to preserve them and fit them for their legitimate work: decaying teeth are a source, as well as a symptom, of disease.

[A] In accordance with a universal law of nature,—"the conservation of energy,"—"gastric juice," upon which digestion depends, "is secreted from the blood by the glands of the stomach, in proportion to the needs of the organism for food, and not in proportion to the amount of food swallowed." There is, therefore, a normal dyspepsia for whatever of excess is taken. Moreover, in such cases, none of the food is well digested.

[B] *Ptyalin*, a vegetable matter contained in healthy saliva, has very peculiar properties: "if mixed with starch and kept at a moderate warm temperature, it turns that starch into grape-sugar. The importance of this operation becomes apparent when one reflects that starch is insoluble, and therefore, as such, useless as nutriment, while the sugar formed from it is highly soluble, and readily oxidizable."—HUXLEY.

Note the special elements tending to insure success in the case of self-treatment just given: The courage, prevalent good temper (so rarely found in these cases), and determination to win (equally rare), did much, very much, toward conquering her disease; but it is more than doubtful if these alone would have sufficed: her success in winning the family over to her radical views, or, at least, in gaining their entire co-operation, was a marked feature looking toward a final victory. None of them ventured to discourage her,—all joined heartily in the work. Had she sat at an ordinary table, one crowded with "good things"; and had her friends persisted in entreating her to eat this, that, and the other thing, it is probable that her good resolutions would have failed, sooner or later,—her life paying the forfeit. And this leads me to mention a most important feature of what has come to be known as the "Salisbury Treatment": "Meals are to be taken at regular intervals, and the patient should eat either alone or with those who are using the same diet, and not sit down at a table where others are indulging in all kinds of food. He should take a good draught—one or two cupfuls—of warm water an hour before each meal; a sponge-bath two or three mornings,[37] and a *comfortable* full bath once a week. For the latter use a little pure Castile soap, but rinse thoroughly. Air-baths and sun-baths are also of great importance. (See 'Air-baths,') Flannel worn next the skin [I should say, that the year round, cotton underwear is far better], and the clothing frequently changed and aired. As much open-air exercise as can be borne without fatigue, or thorough rubbing and pounding of the body [or squeezing of the muscles of the entire body, with a firm grasp of the attendant's hand] morning and evening for those too weak to take exercise."

[37] If desirable, this bath may be taken later in the day; but it should *never* occur within one hour before, nor until at least three hours after any meal. The temperature of the water should be agreeable with sensitive patients, but gradually lowered from day to day, until *cool* water becomes agreeable.

It is the prevalent belief that hot food is desirable especially for feeble persons, inclined to chilliness; but while smoking-hot dishes produce a temporary feeling of warmth and comfort, this is usually succeeded by a "reaction," producing a still greater degree of chilliness: the congestion excited by the presence of the hot food or drink, soon subsides, leaving the stomach anæmic, delaying digestion, perhaps preventing it altogether. Cool food, properly masticated, acquires in the mouth a normal temperature, and thus enters the stomach without producing the unnatural stimulation which arises from the ingestion of hot food, and which is likely, in the case of feeble persons, to cause, secondarily, most mischievous effects. A single mistake of this sort may excite congestion of the lungs, and undo the good work of weeks of right living. This can not seem incredible, in view of the fact that a single excessive meal often excites an attack of congestion of the lungs in the case of robust persons. True, in these instances the disorder is usually attributed to "a sudden cold," whether the victim can or can not recall any exposure, but the fact is as I have stated. I have had many instances like the following: A business man, accustomed to an outdoor life, rises in the morning after a good night's sleep, feeling as well as usual; eats a hearty breakfast, dons his overcoat, walks briskly to his place of business, and entering the *hot, close office*, perhaps within thirty minutes from the time of rising from the breakfast-table, he finds himself so hoarse that he can hardly make himself understood, and feels a pressure at the lungs indicating a great degree of congestion. There is but one way to explain this: a predisposition; a hot meal, rapidly eaten; active exercise taken immediately thereafter, and while the stomach is engorged with food—what more is needed? The wonder is, not that this man is suddenly made sick, but, rather, that he is not oftener so.

The consumptive will often derive great benefit from a full stomach-bath daily, consisting of about a pint of tepid water rapidly swallowed, on rising or an hour before breakfast. This will not create nausea or excite vomiting, unless there is occasion for these symptoms, arising from the presence of undigested food; but it will prove healing, prevent thirst and the necessity for drinking with, or directly after, meals—although, whenever there is thirst, the patient should drink pure cool water, moderately, but to his satisfaction, finally. It is better, however, as a rule, to drink regularly, an hour or so before each meal, such an amount as suffices to *prevent* thirst, while not causing a feeling of discomfort soon after drinking. A little practice, with careful observation, will soon enable the patient to judge how much to take.

OPEN-MOUTH BREATHING.

I am not going to recommend the consumptive, nor any person, well or ill, to do all or much of his breathing through the mouth; on the contrary, I agree that the nostrils were designed to warm and filter the air, and that in general this is necessary. But there are times when the atmosphere does not require to be *filtered* and when it had better not be *warmed*; and I wish to do away with all fear of danger from casual or occasional open-mouth breathing, especially in the *open air*, and in winter, or at any season when there is freedom from dust, and regardless of the weather, and the time of day or night. For "sore" or irritated throat and bronchi, or oppressed lungs, I have found persistent open-mouth breathing of pure cold air curative in its tendency; and have myself, upon occasion, gone out on a winter's night, to walk and breathe in this manner by the hour. Consumptives are often subject to attacks of dyspnœa (difficult breathing), but rarely, if ever, do they come on out of doors; it is rather, when, having been vouchsafed a little pure respiratory food, the lungs are again forced to respire the hot, poisoned, make-believe air of the home, that the congestion takes place. And this may be set down as the only danger in the premises, viz.: the return from the fresh, pure and bracing atmosphere without, to the over-heated and under-ventilated living-rooms. The remedy, then, for an attack under such circumstances would be found in throwing open the doors and windows—keeping well wrapped or warm in bed—rather than in sealing the crevices and piling on fuel. Even *pneumonia*, most dreaded of "diseases," in which the lungs are congested to engorgement, is now being successfully treated on this principle—the persistent open-mouth breathing of out-door air, if in the winter, or the same, drawn through an ice-packed refrigerator—(scrupulously clean and profusely ventilated), if the weather be warm; the patient, meanwhile, being *warm* in bed, though never sweltered with wraps [the aim being to balance the temperature, by cooling the head, heating the feet, and exposing and sponging the feverish surface, as may be indicated], and supplied with a proper face-piece to which is attached a flexible tube, through which the cold air is passed direct to the lungs; this manner of breathing to be *constant* and *uninterrupted*, hour after hour, and throughout the night, if necessary (*never* remittent), until the temperature of the patient, as indicated by the thermometer placed under the arm, is reduced to about the normal point (98.2° F.), and the pressure at the lungs relieved. The philosophy of this treatment is as evident as is that of the playing of an engine upon the hottest part of a fire.

A WORD ABOUT THE BED.

The bed and its covering constitute the night-clothes, and for the bed-ridden patient day-clothes as well. Therefore, we can hardly place too much importance upon the bed and its appointments. And yet, in view of all that has been said relating to cleanliness and wholesomeness, in a general way, but few words are necessary to tell the story. The bed may be of straw, even, and still, if full, fresh, and well-made, be every way sufficient for comfort and health,—better, indeed, than a poor or long-used mattress of any sort;—a mattress of hair, cotton, or wool makes a complete bed. A feather bed is the worst of all. Whatever the bed may be, it should remain open and airing whenever the patient is out of it for any length of time; hence the bed-room should not be the sitting-room when avoidable. Patients confined to the bed altogether, should, if possible, have two—one for day the other for night use—each kept airing during all the time it is unoccupied, and, when practicable, placed in the open air and in the sunshine a portion of the day; the more the better. After the cotton or linen sheets, the covering (of as little weight as is consistent with comfort) should, in place of the common "comfortables," consist of woolen blankets, which, being porous, are less "stifling" to the body (see foot-note, p. 171), and permit of being readily cleansed and dried; and they should be thus treated as often as once in three or four weeks, at least, and oftener if the thorough airing recommended is not given them. The "sick-room" should be the "healthiest" room in the house—bright, sunny, and made as "cheery" as possible. No "long-faces" should enter it; there should be no "croning about"—no constant "how-do-you-feel-to-days," nor subdued looks or airs. Carry along a happy, cheery face and tone, or keep out of the sick-room altogether. Above all, no mind-pictures about eating, eating, eating—unless, the patient is past hope!

THE POSITION IN BED.

As well as when up and about, is a matter of importance to the sick or well. With the sick, the habit of "rounding up" to the disease is every way prejudicial. Consumptives are especially inclined to seek present ease to their ultimate hurt. It should be one of the aims, in "lung difficulties," to increase the breadth of the chest in order to give more room for the expansion of the lungs; and this demands increased efforts to expand the lungs, and to push the shoulders back—gradually, very gradually, never to the extreme, but with steady persistence. No radical and immediate change must be looked for; none can be accomplished, in any direction, whether in the shape of the body, quality of lung tissue, or breathing power; but a gradual transformation may be inaugurated, and ensured by means of persistent effort, as the general health improves. It is best to lie, at least much of the time spent in bed, as nearly flat upon the back as possible, slightly inclining toward the side, or alternating between the two positions, with the head low; arms and legs "at ease," the latter not drawn or "curled" up, but slightly relaxed. If the general regimen is strictly hygienic, the position as thus described will, so far from working any harm, prove of advantage—favoring free breathing, as well as the fullest rest of the body. Where there is shortness of breath and difficulty in breathing, the patient is inclined to cultivate the habit of narrowing the shoulders, and so bolstering himself in bed as to still further shorten the breath, thus temporarily easing the difficulty, but finally increasing the disease. He needs to courageously take the opposite course (never rashly, however), and meet the consequences, which are likely to be manifested in some increase of coughing and raising—the very things he needs to do, but which he is apt to shrink from as much as possible. In avoiding natural "expectorants," the necessity for artificial ones seems to arise. In the one case he raises with some effort what, in his present state, may be described as the normal amount of mucus; in the other, expectoration is easier because there is more to raise. The former is curative; the latter tends to fatality.

Well knowing that sexual indulgence constitutes one of the most fruitful causes of this disease—of decline, in short, however exhibited—I will conclude by saying, that the consumptive should *never* depart from the rule of strict continence. (See Appetite.) No language can exaggerate the importance of this injunction for a person who is even threatened with decline, if he means to eradicate his disease. The sexual and the nervous systems (including the brain) act and react upon one another, keeping both abnormally alert, and these upon the digestive and assimilative, through the sympathetic, altogether making a quadrangular fight well calculated to impair—to break down, indeed—the strongest constitution; while with the less vigorous (often the most lascivious; or, maybe, the victim of a libidinous but otherwise considerate companion) the case is hopeless, unless the true remedy is applied. The patient should sleep alone, if possible, not even the husband or wife sharing the bed—a rule which, from every point of view, is of importance to both the patient and the attendant.

Note.—The underlying principle of this work prohibits the idea of a specific and exclusive treatment for this, that, and the other *disease* mentioned; for these are named simply in order that we may make a beginning toward understanding the term *sickness*: the entire volume, from preface to finis, is a treatise on the origin of sickness, its prevention and cure. In view of this, we can not leave the consumptive here, while the dyspeptic, the rheumatic, or the *douloureux*-tic is invited to a consideration of his peculiar symptoms,—for these, in large measure, are mere accidents, since the rheumatic of to-day may be the paralytic of to-morrow, and the dyspeptic of this year the consumptive next, and so on. But all classes, and all who wish to inform themselves as to what makes pain and sickness, and what ends these symptoms, should study carefully the various chapters, omitting none.

CHAPTER IV.

CONSTIPATION.

Temporary non-action of the bowels as excretory organs, is entirely normal under certain conditions, as (1) following diarrhœa or looseness, whether caused by indigestion or physic, (2) throughout the period of a fast, (3) for the mother, several days (varying from 3 to 10), at confinement,[38] and (4) at such other times as "Nature finds it necessary to muster all the energies of the system for some special purpose, momentarily of paramount importance," as in alarming sicknesses where, accompanied by lack of appetite, the bowels remain closed for a considerable period of time. In none of these circumstances should there be continued efforts to excite action. In the last-named instance the lower bowel may need a clearing out by free injection at the *beginning,* and whenever there are fecal matters to remove; but when convalescence is established, the appetite and strength have returned, food is taken and digested, the bowels will act of their own accord. The practice of forestalling nature in this matter by using physic or injections is often the cause of much mischief—it is an impertinent interference in nature's plans, and is seldom useful. If the sufferer is never fed, except at convalescence and when a *natural appetite* has returned, and then only with plain, wholesome food,—restricting the quantity to the present capacity for digestion and absorption,—the evacuation of the lower bowel may be awaited without any feeling of anxiety or alarm at its seeming tardiness. Returning strength is the only needed physic.

[38] The very common practice of administering purgatives or injections a few days after confinement is not only unnecessary—it is fraught with mischief and often with disaster. I have known of instances where robust women were kept sick, and dangerously so, in bed for weeks in

consequence of the free use of oil administered by the physician (according to his invariable practice) on the third and succeeding days. At her next confinement, one lady who had suffered as above, having lived hygienically during the gestation period, suffered very little pain, was on her feet, washed and dressed her baby, and had a natural movement on the second day. In another case purgation was attempted on the third day and, oil not acting promptly, the total results of profuse injections at intervals for the next three days, was, on the *sixth* day, to bring away about a *teaspoonful of strawberry seeds*, the residue of berries eaten on the previous day. It is evident that the food was well digested and absorbed into the circulation, and that no fecal matters were secreted; hence no occasion for the bowels to "move," in the common understanding of the term. In cases where women approaching confinement are troubled with constipation (entirely unnecessary if they will live properly), the lower bowel should be evacuated by the aid of free injections prior to delivery; but succeeding that event nature may well be left to herself for a time. Nature, however, does not have a fair chance where patients of this class are overfed; hence, and hence only, the necessity for "aiding" her in moving the bowels.

In case of severe constipation, injections—internal baths, so to say—may be employed in emergencies, but infrequently and with extreme care, lest they aggravate the evil and provoke others. Although in no sense as injurious as purgative medicines, which inevitably impair the nutritive organs, still enemas should never be depended on for daily movements. Next to a correct dietary, with liberal exercise in the open air, one of the best aids in promoting regular action of the bowels is, in my opinion, passive exercise—kneading of the bowels for say five minutes or more before each meal—and the more active exercise of, say, imitating for a few minutes the arms-and-body swinging motions of a mower in the hay-field; spending another few minutes in hopping up and down, twice on each foot alternately, while "keeping time" by slapping the thighs and swaying the body to the right and left; stooping and rising, bending forward and back, etc.; twisting the body around, first one way and then the other, with the hips as the pivotal point (at stool this last greatly facilitates the ejective process), etc., etc. Sedentary persons, and all who feel "chilly" at times, will find, upon trial, that a few minutes devoted to such exercise, occasionally, or whenever the need is felt, will be far more satisfactory than extra garments, or hovering about the fire: it sets the blood a-tingling in the veins and warms a body up.[39] (See Consumption, for general regimen as to diet, air, exercise, clothing.) If for a time the bowels are willful in the matter of demanding rest to complete a process of healing going on in the diseased glands when there has been distention and irritation, or until a reformed dietary shall have strengthened the general system when, from any cause, it has been under-nourished, and there is, consequently, no action for two, three, or even four days at a time, it need occasion no alarm, and the novice will be surprised to see how natural a movement will finally reward his or her patience in awaiting the call of nature, instead of badgering her into unnatural activity. It must be remembered that it is *good health that ensures daily movements*, and not *daily movements good health*. Indeed, when produced by hook or crook, as is often the rule with infants, and adults, even, they do much harm. Daily purgations or injections are made necessary only by gross feeding; and if the latter abuse be persisted in it may be best to move the bowels frequently at all hazards. Under the influence of this combination, however, the small intestines are often so disordered as to impair, even destroy, their power of assimilating food, and together with the colon, or large intestine, become so torpid as almost to require the use of dynamite to move them.

[39] William Cullen Bryant,—a most worthy model, mentally, morally, and physically—thus explains how he had "reached a pretty advanced period of life without the usual infirmities of old age." Next to his abstemious and mostly vegetable diet, and pure moral life, we may well agree with him in the belief that his wonderful preservation was largely due to his custom of going to bed early and early rising, and "for a full hour, immediately upon rising, with very little encumbrance of clothing, taking a series of exercises, designed to expand the chest, and at the same time call into action all the muscles and articulations of the body," followed by a bath "from head to foot."—*Hygiene of the Brain*: $1.50[C] New York, M. L. Holbrook.

[C] This most valuable work contains letters from a score or more of eminent men and women who have lived to advanced age, descriptive of their living habits. The similarity of their mode of life is a feature worthy of remark.

STRAINING at stool is, beyond a slight degree, abnormal, or is made necessary only by abnormal conditions, which render defecation difficult; it tends to perpetuate and increase the difficulty, and should not be practiced ordinarily. The congestion and engorgement of the blood-vessels in the region of the rectum and anus from various causes, as retained fecal matters, or irritation and congestion of the genital organs (which two causes act and react upon each other), produce hemorrhoids (piles), and this complaint is aggravated by the straining referred to. In such cases resort must be had to cool or tepid injections for a time. One effect of deep breathing, from either exercise or habit—filling the lungs in such a manner as to press the diaphragm downward—is to cause regular pressure on the bowels, which aids in exciting their vermicular motion, and facilitates the action, both of the small intestines as digesters, and of the lower bowel in its secretory and excretory functions. The "movement," when natural, consists of *waste matters secreted from the blood* by the glands of the colon, and not, as is popularly supposed, of food substances, at least not to any considerable degree. When it does (and I am bound to say that this is the rule, rather than the exception), it is because the person has eaten at least *that much* more than he ought. A good rule for many who suffer tortures of mind because of constipation would be: mind your own business and let your bowels mind theirs. Strive not to *have* movements, but rather to *deserve* them. That is, attend to the general health by living hygienically, and the bowels will, if given *regular opportunity*, move when there is anything to move for! With infants or young children, a little excess of food will, at first, occasion a little looseness, or increased action, usually; deficiency in diet would cause constipation. The remedy in either case is plain: a little less food in the one case, a little more in the other. The first symptom, looseness, could not result from deficiency in diet, that is, if the deficiency related to quantity solely—the quality being plain and digestible. Tanner had no movement during his fast; Griscomb's experience was similar, and Connolly, the consumptive, who fasted forty-three days, had no movement for three weeks, and then the temporary looseness was occasioned by profuse water-drinking, which in his case proved curative. In common life, it is rare indeed that constipation is the result of a deficient diet, although it often arises from lack of nourishment consequent upon excess, or an unwholesome variety of food, or both. Usually it may be regarded as the "reaction" from over-action. The not uncommon experience, in regular order, is this: Excess in diet, diarrhœa, constipation, physic or enema, purgation, worse constipation, more physic, and so on. The term reaction here means simply that the organs involved having been irritated by undigested food, and having by means of increased action cleared away the obstructions, now seek restoration by the most natural method, as the name itself implies—rest. What are commonly called diseases are in reality cures; and the common practice, with drug doctors, of

"CONTROLLING THE SYMPTOMS,"

is like answering the cries and gesticulations of a drowning man with a knock on the head. If when these intestinal disorders arise, or have become serious, their chief cause—over-feeding—be kept up, the next of nature's remedies may be inflammation of stomach or bowels, or both, followed, perhaps, by *dysentery*, which is the most serious phase of constipation. These are very alarming symptoms, and demand entire abstinence from food until they are considerably abated; pure water should be given freely, and, when possible, exercise to some degree in the open air; tepid water injections, followed by gentle kneading of the bowels for a few minutes, occasionally, to promote the circulation in that region, thus favoring the cleansing and healing process. The appearance of a little fresh blood, even, following this treatment, should not excite alarm; on the contrary, it is, *per se*, a favorable symptom. This special phase of the subject is treated more at length in the author's work entitled "How to Feed the Baby."

A very common mistake with the laity, and often enough made by physicians in diagnosing this complaint, is that of considering a comfortable daily movement conclusive proof that the bowels are not constipated. Few people have tongues that are entirely clean, and a coating there indicates, unmistakably, a worse one of the stomach and intestines.[40] The daily—perhaps semi-daily—action is the result of purgation often, though they would scorn the idea of taking physic—the quantity or quality of their food being such as to cause a degree of indigestion and consequent irritation sufficient to produce purgative effects. While this condition can be endured, all seems to be going along well. There is, to be sure, more or less of acidity, sour stomach, eructations of acrid matters (see the Salisbury theory in article on Consumption), flatulence, headache, neuralgic or rheumatic pains—more or less in number of the scores of ailments so common as to be considered almost normal—but not immediately any serious or alarming complaint. But, after a time, longer or shorter, according to the constitution of the individual, the movements become less satisfactory—irregular and not as profuse as common, and are passed with some difficulty, perhaps. Next to the mistake of resorting to drugs in these cases, is the quite common one of swallowing special kinds of food for the same purpose, and there, is some question as to which of the two evils is the least. An excessive quantity of rye mush, wheaten grits, or oat groats, with a generous dressing of butter, syrup, milk, or honey to wash it down in abnormal haste, will often purge the bowels like the most drastic poison. Active exercise in the open air, taken in conjunction with a proper diet, would prove curative; but in default of this the case goes from bad to worse, until in spite of all the efforts made, the constipation becomes more and more obstinate, various symptoms increasing in degree and new ones appearing, until there almost certainly follows a severe "attack" of some sort: whether this be typhoid, bilious, rheumatic, or scarlet fever, erysipelas, diphtheria, or what not, depends upon the age, surroundings, and diathesis of the patient.

[40] See chapter on Consumption.

All such attacks may be called Nature's kill-or-cure remedies when, as a last resort, she is forced to adopt "heroic treatment"; but aid her in the Natural Cure and she is most kind.

NOTE.—Attention is called to the notes following Consumption, and Bright's Disease.

CHAPTER V.

BRIGHT'S DISEASE (ALBUMINURIA).

In its later stages, this is one of the worst forms of disease. It is often said to be caused by "cold." There can be no doubt but what a person whose kidneys are already badly diseased, and, consequently, his whole system depraved, may have a violent illness excited by extreme exposure to wet and cold. The same may be said in case of one reduced by any exhausting form of disease; but sound-bodied men, living hygienically, could never have this disease, whatever the degree of cold they might have to endure. On the contrary, this disease is not known among the residents of the polar regions; our own explorers among the ice-fields of the north do not have it, although exposed for long periods to a temperature at 40° to 60° F. below zero, and to changes of so extreme a character that our temperate climate affords no parallel to them. "In the accounts of Arctic expeditions, though the most intense cold was often endured, under circumstances of great fatigue, by men previously weakened by disease and hardship, this is not among the diseases from which they suffered. Dr. Kane's men, though enduring extreme cold, exposed on one occasion for seventy-two hours at a mean temperature of 41° below zero, suffered fearfully from frost-bite and scurvy, but not from any renal affection. Other travelers within the Arctic circle bear the same testimony, and I have been informed by those familiar with the cold districts of North America, that there renal dropsy is unknown."[41] "The travelers in the frigid zone are exposed to far greater and more sudden transitions of temperature than are ever felt in our changeable but temperate climate. Capt. Parry states that his men often underwent a sudden change of 120°, in passing from the cabin of the vessel to the outer air, and yet none but the most trifling complaints resulted. Here we have all the circumstances from which experience would lead us to anticipate renal disease, viz.: great preceding depression, intense and protracted cold suddenly applied.... Extreme cold," continues Dr. Dickinson (ibid.) "though it may stop cutaneous exhalation, probably does not allow the material that would cause renal inflammation to accumulate. Cold increases the action of oxygen and gives rise to increased combustion of the solids and fluids of the body. This condition, as I have emphasized elsewhere repeatedly, occasions a demand for a large amount of food daily, to supply the waste, and exalts the digestive powers correspondingly. The moral of all this, for those who, living in a temperate climate, would avoid these disorders—all physical disorders, indeed—is that *here the above conditions can not obtain to the extent of rendering possible the digestion* and *absorption* of *three full meals a day*. Only under exceptional circumstances are *two* such meals ever thoroughly digested and assimilated —they can never be, unless needed; and this fact is not disproved simply because inexperts do not recognize the symptoms of indigestion which everywhere prevail among themselves. Some of the most incorrigible workers, with both brain and muscle, known to me, take but *one meal a day*,[42] and this because they found the change necessary in order to enable them to perform their arduous labors and preserve their health. Others similarly situated divide this meal into *two halves*—taking a small meal morning and night, or, better than the latter, a lunch in the morning, and at night, after ample rest, the principal meal. No person ever tried this plan and found any need of a change because of lack of nourishment.[43] I mention this last point to meet the stock objection of people who essay to escape from the logic of the position—the necessity for the modification of their own dietetic habits—behind the old dogma, 'one's meat is another's poison.' (See p. 43.) It is entirely probable that a robust man (a frail one would succumb to the exposure, with or without food) exposed for days together, and for the entire twenty-four hours, to the extreme cold of winter, exercising vigorously meantime, could eat three full meals a day and escape digestive disorder. The habit of approximating as nearly as possible to this diet, in a temperate climate, or while the bodily warmth is maintained by artificial heat, originates the greater proportion of our ailments; while lack of exercise, and the folly of attempting to oxygenate this excessive quantity of food with air that is breathed over and over again—a process which one writer likens to eating one's own fœces—amply accounts for the balance.

[41] "Treatise on Albuminuria," by W. Howship Dickinson, M.D., F.R.C.P., etc., p. 54.

[42] See note on The One-Meal System.

[43] The fact is—and it can not be made too prominent—ninety-nine in the hundred, of all classes of people, eat in excess of their needs, and the "small eater," eating without appetite, eats, relatively speaking, more excessively than the gross-feeder whose appetite never fails.

"By cold the respiratory function is exalted, and the excretion of urea is diminished. With the intense cold of the North Pole (and in the *open air*), the introduction of oxygen by the lungs is probably so great, and the oxidation in the body so active, that all material susceptible of such action becomes oxidized, as much of it as can be converted into carbonic acid passing out with the breath. The kidneys, therefore, are not liable, as in temperate climates, to be irritated by excrementitious matter, for the stress of excretion falls upon the lungs." (Ibid.) The practical question then is, What can we do, in this particular climate, that shall tend to give us exemption from a disease that can not exist at the poles, where the cold is intense enough to require a man to eat all he can, nor at the tropics, when the heat is met with a diet of juicy fruits?[44] (See article on Fruits.) Simply this, and nothing more; so regulate the diet as to forbid indigestion, or, in other words, eat according to our needs, as governed by work and weather; and all that has been said about the cause and prevention of "colds" (see C.) is applicable right here.

[44] Sojourners from the North, at the tropics, are exempt from disease so long as they live on the fruits of the soil; but a beef and brandy regimen makes short work with them.

Winter weather (inoperative, however, for those who spend their time in close, warm rooms), scant clothing, much exercise, fresh air—these conditions, so far as present, and to the extent of a man's subjection to them, require a larger quantity of food than could be digested under opposite conditions, and tend to mitigate the effects of over-indulgence as to amount and quality. In our climate, however, not one person in ten thousand lives, even in the coldest weather, sufficiently under these influences to require the diet necessary at the poles, viz., three full meals of mixed food, largely composed of fat. Hence, the only palliatives a person can resort to, who adheres to the prevalent mode of living, as to diet, are those conditions that approach as nearly as possible to those obtaining in the frigid zone; but these conditions can not be, at least are not, enjoyed here, to a point rendering exemption from disease possible even for the most robust. But when we reflect upon the fact that our people are not, as a rule, robust (although this would be otherwise but for the unbalanced circumstances under consideration), that they live in warm rooms, wear heavy clothing even within doors, and don thick wraps on going out, work as little as possible (all tending to the need of abstemiousness), and that in the face of all this they do not, at least to any appreciable extent, voluntarily restrict their appetites, but do, in fact, even in summer, imitate the blubber-eaters of the North, nearer than they do the fruit-eaters of the South; that Sabbath morning finds the New Englander, for example, gorging himself with pork and beans, hot brown bread dripping with butter, hot, strong coffee, etc.; Tuesday, roast-beef, with plenty of gravy; Wednesday—"boiled mutton, with caper sauce," and so on to Saturday's boiled dinner, of corned-beef, greasy cabbage, etc. (the diet of the poor differing chiefly in the quality, or price per pound), and this just the same during the warmest week in winter as during the coldest, and regardless of any of the possibly varying circumstances, as hard work out of doors, or light work, or none at all, within; and that this same folly runs into and becomes greater folly in the spring and summer even, except so far as nausea or lack of appetite cause an involuntary modification,—in view of all this we need not look altogether, nor indeed at all, to heredity to account for the wretched disorders to which we, as a people, are subject, and which prevail to an extent almost transforming our literary and art periodicals into indirect partnership-relations with the manufacturers of quack "remedies" for all forms of sickness; this class of advertisers *pay* too liberally to exclude their flaunting lies. I look almost in vain for even a religious journal that refuses to devote any portion of its space to medical advertisements. Do our religious editors themselves believe in, and take, the "pills" they advertise?

Bright's Disease is one that never attacks those who live on coarse food, live abstemiously, and drink water chiefly. It is rather a disease of "high livers." But a man does not need a large income to ensure this affection: any one who can get all he wants to eat and drink, and who eats and drinks all he "wants" (even without indulgence in wine, or alcohol in any form, which is a prolific cause of this disorder), may safely reckon on some of the symptoms, if not upon the worst form of the disease; and whether it be the understood cause of his death or not, it will surely be a contributing cause. The possession of typically healthy kidneys is a rare circumstance in this climate. The excessive micturition so universal in infancy, occasioned by excess in diet, is the beginning of renal disease.

Dr. Bright immortalized his name by discovering the fact that, when a man's last sickness is attended with a certain class of symptoms, as albumen in the urine, final suppression of the urine, and uremic poisoning, they are occasioned by a peculiar disease or degeneration of the kidney. From a practical stand-point we care nothing about the kind of change taking place in the kidney, but rather ask what kind of change in our habits will keep this, and all the organs of the body, in a healthy condition? The former study is all well enough for those who desire it, but if *too much time* is devoted to it, and to the *relation of drugs thereto*, by an individual, he may be, probably will be, the very least fitted to advise an inquirer who desires to know what he can do to be saved from disease and the supposed necessity of taking medicine. Says Dr. Dickinson (ibid., chap. VI.): "There are few disorders which are more under the influence of medicine than is the catarrhal inflammation of the kidneys." And the very next sentence is one worth pondering on by those who are accustomed to take medicine whenever they come to grief through ignorance or neglect of the laws of life: "Under some plans of treatment," says this celebrated authority, in continuing, "plans which formerly were almost universally adopted, and *still have their advocates*, the disorder is one of heavy mortality. Under other circumstances the danger is so small, that if once the complaint be recognized, a recovery may be reckoned upon in a large *proportion* of cases. Without treatment of any kind there is reason to suppose that a large *majority* of the subjects of it would recover." (The italics are my own.) From this it will be observed that it depends on one's luck whether he shall fall into the hands of a practitioner who belongs to a class still adhering to the plan ensuring a "heavy mortality," or of one whose modified form of treatment is less fatal; and upon his good sense, whether he shall come under the influence of either, or adopt the methods indicated herein, viz., the abandonment of disease-producing, and the adoption of *ease*-producing, habits, which would be an immense gain over the "no treatment" plan which, according to a rational interpretation of Dr. Dickinson's language, is the safest of the three referred to by him. From the three-hundred-page treatise before me, which is fresh from the mint (1881), and is a most valuable book for those who wish to study the pathology of the disease (Bright's), but which is little calculated to aid any one healthward, except he be already pretty well informed in hygienic matters, I cull, in addition to the paragraphs already quoted, the following little nugget of pure gold: "We must avoid the use of any drugs which, under the name of stimulating diuretics, might exasperate the existing congestion; and we must enforce such diet as to reduce to a minimum that nitrogenous excess which finds its way out chiefly by the kidneys, and provides in many shapes effective means of irritation. Physiological repose is to be sought, not by debarring the gland of the harmless and necessary solvent, but by cutting off the materials of urea and uric acid." How naturally, then, do we look for the continuing sentiments: "'Spare diet and spring water clear' may often be found sufficient though simple remedies. *Of all diuretics water is the best.*"[45] But how can we reconcile, with such counsel, the treatment that he himself commonly adopts?

[45] Ibid., p. 86. The italics are my own, and I am amazed to find that this best diuretic is rarely the one used, and never fairly tested by this authority, who seems almost to exhaust the *materia medica* in the treatment of even infants of tender age.

In one case noted by him, and in which, as he says, "the attack was slight," and "the boy became convalescent," but later, although under the doctor's own eye at the hospital, with "no evidence of his having taken cold," he became worse, went on to a fatal termination, "the urine becoming loaded with albumen and abounding with fibrinous casts—convulsive attacks—death!" It seems to me easy enough, however, to reconcile the unfavorable turn and the fatal termination with the treatment he adopted, viz., digitalis instead of "the best diuretic" (water); "fluid diet," consisting chiefly of beef-tea—a non-nutritive fluid whose solid constituents are mainly urea, kreatine, kreatinine, isoline, and decomposed hæmatine, exactly the animal constituents of the urine, except that there is but a trace of urea.[46]

[46] London *Lancet*.

As the little fellow grew worse, "a little brandy was given to counteract the depressing effect of the digitalis." "On the 27th, the pulse had fallen to 52, and was not quite regular; the brandy was therefore increased to two ounces daily," with digitalis every six hours; later, a "diuretic draught composed of scoparium, acetate of potash, and nitric ether; on the 29th, this diuretic mixture was changed by the addition of nitre and squills; on the 30th, as was anticipated, he was seized with eliptiform convulsions, a succession of which came on, accompanied with foaming and biting of the tongue, and caused his death in two hours and a half."[47] The next case reported was that of a child eighteen months old, treated at the hospital by the same physician, and described: "Dropsy—persistent diarrhœa—peritonitis—death." "The child," says the celebrated practitioner and author, "was frequently fed with pounded meat and milk; a little brandy was given, and opiates and astringents were prescribed to check the diarrhœa." As he went on to his fate, he was made to swallow the following remedies: "opium, dilute sulphuric acid, tincture of the sesquioxide of iron, acetate of lead. The quantity of brandy was increased to three ounces daily.

The child became paler and had a sunken look," etc. "The child sunk a week after admission." I make mention of these cases for the reason that up to this day the same horrible treatment is being practiced. Although these, and many even worse cases contained in this new work, transpired some years ago and were recorded in the first edition, still they remain in the new edition unaccompanied by any note of warning; and young or old medical students pore over and imitate the examples here set before them.

[47] The case of Thomas Vallance, 9 years old. Oh, wise physician: the fatal symptoms came along "as anticipated!"

I quote another paragraph from the treatise of Dr. Dickinson, which, if it has, as would seem evident, thrown little light about the doctor's own pathway, as regards the appropriate treatment of the disorder, will prove instructive to some of my readers, and bear favorably upon my theory of disease. In the early pages (p. 29) of the treatise, Dr. Dickinson says: "It may be generally stated that this inflammatory disease arises from unnatural stimulation of the kidneys. The blood is charged with [food] material excessive in quantity or unnatural in quality, which these glands take upon themselves to remove. Their own proper elements of secretion are poured upon them in sudden and excessive amount, or matter is thrown upon them which is foreign to their usual habit. As a consequence of overwork, or of work to which they are not adapted, they take on a turbulent and abnormal activity. They become congested, the tubes get choked up with epithelial growth, and the disease is established."

Many of the symptoms in the following list are more or less frequently, some of them invariably, present in the case of supposably healthy infants, and are commonly considered as entirely normal. Fairly considered, however, they are the effects of excess in diet. To the greatest possible extent the superfluous water contained in their gross diet passes off by the kidneys, causing immediately a diseased condition of those organs from overwork; the cellular tissue becomes loaded and distended with the fatty matters, and also with much water, unrecognized as dropsy until it reaches immense proportions; what really amounts to purging is so universal as to be regarded as the normal state of an infant's bowels, and this is, sooner or later, often very early, succeeded by the reaction termed constipation. The back-aching that results from all this is none the less terrible because the little sufferers can not talk and tell where the pain is; peevishness, general *malaise*, and crying, tell of suffering, not of (their) perversity. Among the

SYMPTOMS OF KIDNEY DISEASE

are the following: frequent and copious micturition (wetting the bed or getting up at night); later the excretion of urine is scant, passed frequently, or, may be, suppressed altogether. Fat; later—emaciation. Heat and dull pain in the loins[48] (small of the back), increased by pressure; slight or considerable "puffing" about the eyes, noticeable only at times, or it may be constant and unrecognized as a symptom of disease; it may be diminished at times, as the secretion of urine becomes modified, or the condition of the system happens, temporarily, to improve. And it increases often when the secretion of urine diminishes, or is passed less freely. The countenance is more or less pallid, and may have a brownish tinge. Croupy breathing accompanies œdema of the larynx. "With children, inflammation of one or other of the organs of respiration is the most fatal tendency of the disease. Not only are they liable to pleurisy, pneumonia, and bronchitis, but, also, to membranous croup." Constant tendency to irritability of manner, easily angered, unreasonableness, petulance; with infants—constant fretting, crying, nothing will interest or amuse them.

[48] Of all portions of the body, this should be lightly covered, never sweltered with wraps, bindings, or weight of garments.

Diphtheria is, I believe, only a phase of albuminuria. Says Dr. Grasmuck, treating of diphtheria, and other physicians have observed the fact: "Another peculiarity of the scourge is its fondness for children of a certain condition—the fat, sleek, soft, tender, 'well-fed' children so generally admired—such children can offer but slight resistance to this disease; being, in fact, chronically diseased, they are predisposed to 'attacks' of all kinds; and, living to adult age, furnish the greater proportion of cases of tuberculous disease. On the other hand," he continues, "I do not know of a single instance where the disease proved fatal to—rarely attacking—a child of the *genus* 'Street Arab'—children who spend most of their time out of doors, are thinly clad, sleep in cold rooms, have a spare diet, and who have no one to pamper them unwisely."

Dr. Dickinson treats of albuminuria under three heads, viz., tubular nephritis, granular degeneration, and lardaceous disease. He designates, also, such other diseases as are likely to result in consequence of this disorder; and finds some of these peculiar to, or more apt to afflict, sufferers from one or the other forms. He says: "It is seen (from the table presented) that nephritis is a disease of infancy and youth, causing most deaths in the first decade coincidentally with the prevalence of scarlatina; many in the third when the toils and exposures of active life are perhaps the most prolific of evil. Granular degeneration belongs to middle and advancing life, and is most fatal between fifty and sixty. The one flourishes upon the febrile accidents [!] of childhood and the susceptibilities of youth; the other develops when *the habits of life begin to tell* and the effects of old age begin to appear. The lardaceous disorder has little to do with either extreme of the mortal course; it is chiefly associated with the *vices of early maturity*, and with tubercle and struma, disorders more incident to the young than the old, and in their suppurative form to youth rather than childhood." Among the diseases resulting, or likely to result, from one or other forms of the disease, Dr. Dickinson names the following: dropsy, pneumonia, pleurisy, peritonitis, bronchitis [before mentioned]; pericarditis, endocarditis, hypertrophy of the heart, with cardio-vascular thickening, [heart "diseases"]; hemorrhagic accidents [bursting of blood-vessels—apoplexy] depending as they do upon structural changes of the vessels; diarrhœa.

SOME OTHER SYMPTOMS.

Nasal catarrh; the radical suppression of this discharge is likely to be followed by serious if not fatal kidney disease.[49] (To remove the former by removing its cause, thus rendering the discharge unnecessary, is quite another thing). Hence the danger of using so-called catarrh remedies, or of adopting any specific local treatment: they are either inert or injurious.

[49] As illustrating this point I will mention the case of M. K., of Troy, N. Y.,—a case of successful (?) self-treatment for catarrh. This patient had for a dozen or more years suffered with nasal catarrh, and had tried most of the advertised "specifics" without avail; in fact, the disorder steadily increased. At last, the twice daily snuffing of slightly soapy water, for some weeks, "cured" him, as he said; but simultaneously with the suppression of the catarrhal discharge there resulted (without, however, any thought of connecting the two events, in the mind of the patient) an excessive flow of urine, extreme thirst, etc., etc.; in short, true diabetes. In this case great relief was experienced from an exclusive diet of skim-milk for five months, the patient swallowing nothing else for that length of time, except two tablespoonfuls, daily, of wheat-bran thoroughly chewed, "for the bowels." At the end of the five months the patient weighed 210 lbs. This he realized as excessive, and my attention being directed to the case at this point, the patient at my suggestion adopted the bread and fruit diet—discontinuing the skim-milk and bran—and gradually reducing his weight by moderate diet and increased exercise, went on to a complete recovery.

Erysipelatous inflammation of the dropsical limbs; "vomiting may happen at any stage, even the earliest; it is often incontrollable." Head symptoms, which occur in the more prolonged forms of the complaint, are usually of a convulsive kind, whereas, in acute cases, coma is apt to set in without any such prelude. Epileptic seizures may be preceded by pain in the head, drowsiness, or peculiarity of manner, or may occur without any premonitory sign.

Says Dr. Dickinson: "The gouty habit, from whatever circumstance it arise, is one of the more obvious and immediate conditions to which granular disease of the kidneys can be traced." ... "The disease is a frequent result of gout; this is by far the most important fact in its etiology. It is one of the results of the gouty diathesis (see Rheumatism), and may precede or follow the external manifestations.... It is scarcely necessary to insist ... that the gouty condition comes first." The fact is that there is a process of degeneration going on throughout the entire structure of the man, even to the last tissue, and the symptoms are all indicative of this; and this is more or less strictly true of all disorders. The naming and classifying of "diseases" is calculated to mystify and mislead: sickness is the proper term for describing them all; self-abuse, in the broadest sense of the word, is the cause of them; and obedience to law, the only means of prevention or cure.

I hold that the gouty, the rheumatic, the strumous, the "colds," and all other diatheses, are practically unimportant distinctions. The technical difference is, of course, well understood and admitted. In any event, it is certain that the course of living best suited to prevent one, is also best adapted to prevent or remove all. For all practical purposes, however, they may be classed together; and whoever desires, either for themselves or their children, exemption from, or the alleviation of, suffering, have only to adopt a pure mode of living in order to escape, or emerge from, the *disease diathesis*.

NOTE.—The limits of this work forbid an extended consideration of the influence of this or that occupation in promoting this disease; nor is it, in my estimation, essential. The trades must go on, regardless of their influence upon health. There must, for example, be painters, plumbers, compositors, tin-workers, etc., even though the absorption of lead does tend to produce the gouty condition and, so, a predisposition to renal disease. A sufficient degree of care in other directions would enable this class to outlive the more favored ones who neglect the laws of life.

See note 2 in Appendix, p. 276.

CHAPTER VI.

INSOMNIA—INSANITY.

Sleeplessness is often referred to as a cause of insanity, but it would be much nearer the truth to say that insanity causes sleeplessness. Dr. Rush says: "A dream is a transient paroxysm of delirium, and delirium a perpetual dream." Not every dreamer becomes insane, in the common understanding of the term, nor every person who is distressed by wakefulness; nor do all those persons who dream dreams of a strange, droll, startling, heart-rending, exhausting character, become inmates of lunatic asylums, although all such are fit subjects for a rigid hygiene; and not a few out of this large number of bad dreamers—who are likewise afflicted with insomnia—but could with advantage place themselves under the charge of an expert in diseases of the brain, or even in an asylum, if either the former, or the physicians in charge of the latter, were in all regards thoroughly equipped for their work—a rare circumstance indeed. Normal sleep is dreamless; in default of this total oblivion, sleep is only partial—it is not perfect nervous repose. No person who suffers severely from indigestion but is also troubled with much dreaming, and, more or less, with wakefulness; and no person who has these last-named symptoms but can safely set them down; at least in great measure, to digestive disorder; and as, almost invariably, removable by improved habits.

Some very wise men have stated as their belief, that no man living is really of sound mind, any more than of sound body, in the strictest application of the term; all have their crazy aspects—their "weak spots," as we say; and the anxious, brooding man, who fears the loss of his reason, may take courage from the thought that his symptoms are only a little worse than his neighbor's, and only demand of him to diminish his dyspepsia if he would become normally insane! To attack insomnia as a disease instead of a symptom, is sure to result in discomfiture in the great majority of cases, and is in every instance unsound in principle. Once established, this condition of wakefulness tends to perpetuate itself; but this would be otherwise with an absolutely natural regimen. A man is wakeful at night because under his present physical condition he ought to be—just as in diarrhœa, the looseness is doing its work of cure. So with all symptoms. *Pain* has its office, and this is coming to be better understood; is already well known to thoughtful, well-informed people; and the *wakefulness* of which so many complain, and which, in some cases, is of the most distressing, painful character, is as truly normal, considering the present physical state of the sufferer's brain, as is pain following a cut. As an aid in the removal of this symptom, next to a radical reform in one's living habits, which is the only possible cure for the disease, the above reasoning is one of the most effectual.

When a man is wounded severely his anxiety is not increased by the pain; it causes no additional alarm, because he knows that it is entirely natural; let him know that sleeplessness is an analogue of pain, and he will, or may, bear it philosophically, and thus tend to its removal. He has a poverty-stricken mind, indeed, who can not, under such circumstances, pass an hour, or several of them, in comparative comfort, knowing that sleep will come in good time. But, thinking all the while that it is sleep only that he needs, his sleeplessness distresses him, causes him to be more and more alarmed, and, consequently, has the effect to postpone the oblivion so devoutly prayed for, but so little earned. To *deserve* sleep is to *have* it. Let the insomniac read the concluding article of this volume, and by the light of it review the hints on diet, air, exercise, etc., in the body of the article on consumption, so as to know what he has to do to become a *good man*, physiologically; and go to bed at about the same hour every night, if possible, or at any rate when he does lie down to sleep it should be after a quiet hour or half-hour devoted to peaceful and thought-steadying occupations, never exciting mental exercise, whether amusing or instructive; and when he draws the blankets about him, let it be with a sublime indifference as to whether he shall or shall not go to sleep promptly. "As to the subduing of the senses, the attempt to shut out external impressions by deafening the ears, closing the eyes, and lowering the sensibilities generally, is in itself a frequently recognizable and always possible cause of persistent wakefulness. The effort to compose the mind (after lying down) and subdue the activity of the senses is made by the higher mental faculty, a part or function of the organism which, of all others, needs to be itself restful in order that the physico-mental being may sleep. It is, therefore, obvious that an *endeavor* to go to sleep is a mistake."[50]

[50] J. Mortimore Granville, M.D., in *Good Words*.

Rather let me, when staring out into the darkness,—for to attempt to shut out the sense of sight by closing the eyes is always to render the inner-mental sense increasingly acute: "the field of sight is soon crowded with grotesque and rapidly changing images—a phantasmagoria, the worrying effect of which is only a too familiar experience of the sleep waiter," and all the mental senses are in like manner stimulated, and their acuteness intensified, by the endeavor to lower the sensibility of the sense organs; and, worst of all, to narcotize them with drugs or sleeping-draughts is irrational and its effects injurious, and if long continued, fatal;—rather, I repeat, having ears to hear, let me hear, and eyes to see, see; and a brain, let me think. Let the brain, the ears, and the eyes "forget their cunning," only when the eyelids droop in sleep because I am sleepy. Meantime, not self-abasingly, but calmly and dispassionately, would I philosophize thus: Well, I am in for it again! I would like to sleep promptly, soundly, and long; why do I not? I suspect that I am not running this physico-mental machine even in a fairly physiological manner; I cause it to run at an abnormal rate during the day, and keep up intense mental excitement through stimulation of one sort or another, prolonging excessive mental activity too far on toward the night; and because of this, and the lack of a fair degree of muscular exercise, I only half breathe; of my fifteen or sixteen inspirations per minute, not one distends the air cells of my lungs to half their capacity. [Thus it transpires that the organism suffers in two ways, viz.: (1) the circulation is not sufficiently oxygenated for its general purposes; and (2) the waste matters are not *"pumped out"* of the substance of the brain,[51] as effectually as need be]. My coffee was strong and nice this morning; it stimulated me very satisfactorily throughout the day; and, what I had not bargained for, I am still feeling the spur (see article on Coffee). That new brand of cigars is exquisitely flavored; but, upon the whole, a perfect night's sleep would be far more exquisite; at least, just now I am in the mood to think so. I sneered at that food-reformer who told me he was never a good sleeper until his present simple, natural habits made him so; but now, just at this moment, it seems as if it would be a good trade to exchange some of my favorite dishes for coarse food and balmy sleep! Oh, if I only could get "balmy" that way every night! I "got the best" of —— yesterday morning on those —— stocks, and spent an hour, bent over my desk, figuring to see how I could get hold of some more at that price, before its holders had time to ascertain its real value. I will tell the widow —— in the morning, what it is worth, instead of trying to buy hers under-price as I contemplated doing. And so I would con over and look through myself and my habits, feeling sure that my eyelids would droop, and sleep would come before I should have completed the work of reform; and I am sure that every sufferer will find that a real reform—a permanent reform—will unfailingly lead on to *health*, and so to sweet and satisfactory sleep.

[51] "As stimulation of the brain causes dilatation of its vessels, and increases the flow of blood through them, mental action of itself not only attracts more blood to the brain, but provides to some extent for the removal of waste products. Hence sleeplessness is normal for a clogged brain. The movements induced by the cardiac pulsations are not so extensive as those caused by the respiratory movements or by muscular exertion, and therefore, when the brain is overworked and the respiratory and muscular movements are restricted, the cerebral nutrition will be diminished by the imperfect removal of waste from its substance. But if, in addition to this, the cerebral cells and fibers are actually poisoned by the circulation within the vessels which supply them, of noxious substances due to imperfect digestion or assimilation, matters will become very much worse."—T. L. BRUNTON, M.D., F.R.S. (ibid.)

"Let no sleepless person be discouraged. Maintain hope under all circumstances. Remember that there are many worse cases of suffering than your own in the world, although to you it seems impossible. Keep up your general health by all sanitary means possible; walk much in the open air, if you can walk; ride, if you can not walk. Above all measures, keep the functions of the skin in prime condition; cleanliness is antagonistic to sleeplessness. Dry friction over the body by the use of the hand, or better by the use of the French hair mitten, twice a day, we have found of great service. The air-bath should not be neglected. A few minutes after the employment of friction over the body, walk about without clothing in a cool room, and if possible let the sun strike upon the body. Do not remain uncovered too long, so as to become chilled. Keep the digestion good; eat only such forms of food as suit the digestive organs. Surround yourself with cheerful company if possible, read such books as do not tax or weary the mind, and life will cease to be a burden, even if you do not sleep as others do. Avoid above all things constant dosing; throw into the ditch, or into the sea, all nostrums that may fall into your hand."

Comparatively few, even of the so-called hopelessly insane, but might in the early stages of their disease be completely restored; and at any period, so long as there is great vital force, or what would commonly pass for robust physical health, no case need be set down as hopeless. But while the present system of treatment prevails (it is not worthy the appellation of "system,") the present small proportion of "cures" will continue to be the rule. The inmates are confined more or less closely, often in imperfectly ventilated apartments, deprived of the exercise in the open air they so much need, to the lack of which in their own homes is, in part, attributable their present condition; they are fed generously, even to plethora; and this, through the fault of the ignorance of their attending physicians, although, if these were wise enough to know when and how their patients needed "dieting," the friends of these sufferers would never submit to anything bordering upon a strictly abstemious diet in their treatment. In visiting lunatic asylums in this and other countries, I have been struck with the appearance of groups of patients—the similarity of their *physique*, as compared with the men and women seen on our streets every day—fat or lean, seldom medium—all exhibiting clearly the physical characteristics of disease, as emaciation, obesity, lack of, or ravenous, appetite, usually the latter. Meal-time comes every five or six hours, and if the appetite is good, all are permitted to eat very much in excess of their needs; they are urged to eat when they desire to fast; and food is forced into their stomachs if they are inclined to abstain for any length of time. It is not uncommon to find patients who upon entering an asylum begin to fatten, though already in an abnormal condition in this regard, their symptoms becoming more and more discouraging as their weight increases, although neither physician nor friends connect the two facts in any way. The latter feel thankful that "poor dear J—— gets enough to eat!" In this connection I introduce an incident of recent occurrence, not as indicating that a compulsory fast for an extended period should be resorted to generally, nor my own belief that it is a specific for all mind-troubles, by any means, but as a fact of great significance which all interested in this question may well pause a moment to contemplate.

[Dispatch from Philadelphia to the New York *Herald*].

TANNER'S RECORD BEATEN.

AN INSANE ASYLUM PATIENT ABSTAINS FROM FOOD FOR FORTY-ONE DAYS.

One of the most extraordinary cases of an insane man attempting to restore his reason by voluntary starvation was discovered recently at the —— County Insane Asylum. The case presents an interesting study for medical men generally. ——, aged forty years, a well-known resident of ——, who has been confined in the institution for the last two years, has abstained absolutely from all food except water, for the space of forty-one days. From the forty-second day of his fast until the fifty-first day he drank one pint of milk daily, and from then began eating strawberries and milk. This diet was maintained for three weeks, and was then succeeded by oatmeal gruel and milk. The case is a matter of careful record at the institution and under circumstances that prevented deception. Therefore, there is not the slightest doubt as to the extraordinary performance having been genuine. Mr. ——, when he first came to the asylum, was very violent at times, but, like many insane persons, he was a ravenous eater. His insanity is supposed to be hereditary. Occasionally he has had lucid intervals, and during these brief periods he frequently expressed the belief that there existed some method by which the insane might have their affliction alleviated if not entirely done away with. To Mrs. ——, the matron of the asylum, he took a great fancy, and, while averse to having anything to do with any other of the officials, he confided in her thoroughly and often expressed the wish that his mind might be restored to him and that he could be released. "For forty-one days," said Mrs. ——, "nothing passed his lips but water, and tepid water at that. Of this fact I am thoroughly positive, knowing as I do the continuous efforts made every day to induce him to eat. When he began the fast he had been living on the same diet as the rest of the patients. He came to me and said, seemingly in a perfectly rational manner, that he was anxious to be cured, and that he thought abstinence from food for a time might benefit him. Mr. —— said he did not intend to carry his experiment to extremes, but that the moment he felt it would be proper for him to break the fast he would do so. On the second day —— again refused to eat, and did not go out of his room. On the third day he drank a small cupful of water. At the end of the seventh day he had drank about six pints of water, and the natural functions of the body had then ceased. All of the attendants were instructed to use every possible means to induce the man to partake of nourishment, and a man was with him constantly through the day."

"Could he not have obtained food at night?" was asked.

"It would have been impossible," replied Mrs. ——. "All the rooms are locked, and none of the patients have access to other parts of the building after sundown. We would have been only too glad had he taken food. About the 20th day he began to get thin and haggard-looking about the face, and seemed to be feeble. He said that his head felt better, and that he did not intend to eat anything as long as he felt so well. On the 35th day he became so weak that he had to go to bed, and remained there until he broke the fast. I had told him that whenever he wanted to eat to send me word, no matter what hour of the night or day it happened to be, and I would see that he was provided with anything he might fancy. On the afternoon of the 41st day since Mr. —— had ceased eating," continued Mrs. ——, "he sent up word by an attendant that he should like to have a cup of coffee.[52] I hastened to comply with the request at once, and had a cup of very strong Java prepared. Mr. —— drank it, and followed it up an hour later with a cup of nice, rich milk. He stuck to the milk for a week, I think, and then added strawberries. This low diet was kept up, oh, for a long time, probably a month, then he gradually began eating oatmeal mush and gruel, which has been maintained up to to-day."

[52] One of the worst moves be could have made; but it is significant that this was his last attempt to return to his coffee habit. In his renewed state it proved no longer enticing!

"And you are perfectly positive, Mrs. ——, that Mr. —— fasted absolutely, with the exception of water, for forty-one days?"

"Perfectly satisfied," replied Mrs. ——; "in fact, I know it. There can be no possible doubt, inasmuch as the attendants were only too anxious to force the man to eat."

"Do you think the fast has made any change in Mr. ——'s condition?"

"Well," replied Mrs. ——, "he will probably be discharged as cured at the next meeting of the board of freeholders in August."[53]

[53] It is a matter of regret to me that this book goes to press before I can ascertain the final result. Judging from the above account, however, I should expect a thoroughly successful ending, unless it should transpire that, true to their instincts, the attendants prevailed upon the patient to abandon the simple regimen, which he adopted after the fast, and resume the ordinary stimulating diet; in which case I should confidently expect a complete relapse.

As a hint regarding the effect of a stimulating and excessive diet upon persons of unsound mind, I subjoin a brief note taken during the trial of the most celebrated lunatic of modern times: "Guiteau's appetite is quite as remarkable as his insolence. He has breakfast served in his room at the court-house about nine o'clock, and usually consumes at this meal a pound of steak, nine buckwheat cakes, three roasted potatoes, and five cups of coffee. Then, at half-past twelve, he gorges himself on roast beef and mutton."

A certain class of wakeful patients are benefited by the practice of eating shortly before bedtime, when this right has been earned by sufficient restriction during the day. To make this the fourth, or even the third meal, however, is almost certain to increase the difficulty at last. The victim of sleepless nights often finds himself quite overcome with drowsiness after his midday meal. If then he could throw himself upon the bed he would have no time to "count," or even think of such a device for putting himself to sleep. He was wide awake before lunch, and but for the habit of taking it, could have finished the day better without than with this out-of-season sleeping potion. Let him take the hint, eat his second and last meal, a sufficient one of plain food, in the evening after fully rested, and, thus equipped, go to bed directly, or after an hour or two of agreeable, but non-taxing, social converse. He must avoid every form of artificial stimulation—tea, coffee, wine, beer, tobacco. To breathe the atmosphere of an office, hotel, or smoking-car, for any considerable period, is no better, may be worse, than a moderate indulgence at first-hand in the open air.

CHAPTER VII.

RHEUMATISM, FATTY DEGENERATION, ETC.

Casey A. Wood. M.D., Professor of Chemistry in the Medical Department of Bishop's College, Montreal, in an article entitled "Starvation in the Treatment of Acute Articular Rheumatism" (Canada *Medical Record*), gives the history of seven cases where the patients were speedily restored to health by simply abstaining from food from four to eight days, and he says he could have given the history of forty more from his own practice, but thought these would suffice. In no instance did he find it necessary to extend the fast beyond ten days. His patients were allowed to drink freely of cold water, or lemonade in moderate quantities, if they preferred, and simple sponging with tepid water was resorted to when indicated by feverishness of the surface. In no case did this treatment fail. No medicine was administered. The cases reported "included men and women of different ages, temperaments, occupations, and social positions." He further says: "From the quick and almost invariably good results to be obtained by simple abstinence from food, I am inclined to the idea that rheumatism is, after all, only a phase of indigestion, and that, by giving complete and continued rest to all the viscera that take any part in the process of digestion, the disease, is attacked *in ipsa radice*." In chronic rheumatism he obtained less positive results, but did not venture to try fasts of longer duration. Dr. Wood concludes by saying that "this treatment, obviating as it does, almost entirely, the danger of cardiac complications, will be found to realize all that has been claimed for it—a simple, reliable remedy for a disease that has long baffled the physician's skill; and the frequency with which rheumatism occurs will give every one a chance of trying its efficacy." As elsewhere remarked, nearly all patients continue eating regularly, until food becomes actually disagreeable, even loathsome, often; and, after this, every effort is exhausted to produce some toothsome compound to "tempt the appetite." Furthermore, and often worst of all, after the entire failure of this programme, the patient can, and usually does, take to gruel or some sort of "extract," which he can drink by holding his breath. All this tends to aggravate the acute symptoms, and to fasten the disease in a chronic form upon the rheumatic patient, or to insure rheumatic fever; and the same principle holds in nearly all acute disorders, it is well to remember. So inveterate is this mania for eating, even when to continue is like turning coals upon the dead ashes and clinkers of an expired fire, that, in ordinary practice, it is well-nigh impossible to induce any class of patients to abstain from food at the beginning of an attack, or to give the fasting cure a fair trial at any stage of the disease. The term frequently applied—"starvation cure"—is both misleading and disheartening to the patient: in fact, he is both *starved* and *poisoned* by *eating* when the hope of digestion and assimilation is prohibited, as is, in great measure, the case in all acute attacks, and more especially when there is nausea or lack of appetite; and he can only escape from the danger by abstaining temporarily. Dr. Wood's prestige in the natural treatment of acute rheumatism was obtained in hospital practice, where it is comparatively easy to "control the symptoms" by withholding the cause, or, in other words, where the physician—providing the nurse is honest—can regulate the diet of his patients, absolutely. After such experience, it was less difficult for Dr. Wood to introduce this remedy among the most intelligent of his patients in private practice; for he could recommend it as in no sense an experiment, but as a remedy of positive advantage and, in fact, indispensable, if the best results were to be effected. My own experience, so far as it goes, has been similar to that of Dr. Wood. Moreover, in chronic cases—cases of long standing—the best results may be hoped for—in fact the best possible results have invariably followed—from an abstemious (*frugivorous*) diet, together with simple bathing, as special symptoms may indicate,—and an improved general regimen, as to fresh air, exercise (inaugurated gradually), beginning, perhaps, with passive exercise, as rubbing, etc., by the attendant. A chronic disease usually implies chronic provocation: Nature has simply commuted the extreme penalty of the law; or, it may be likened to the reprieve of a convict under sentence of death, with an assurance of full liberty upon complete reform.

Among the disorders radically and safely removed by fasting, is

OBESITY,

or any degree of excess in weight. Time, from ten days up. The weight, in this disorder, will diminish under the influence of fasting—by the waste and excretion of *material that can best be spared* (fat)—at the rate of from one to three pounds, or more, a day, which rate of progress can be increased, happily, by exercise in the open air. Entire abstinence from food will cause the fat to disappear, but there can be no regeneration of the muscular system—on the contrary, it must continue to deteriorate—without exercise. It is better, therefore, to keep up a good degree of exercise, and to eat a limited amount of food daily. It is not that the fat person eats or digests more than the lean one (he may not eat nearly as much in fact), but he excretes less. Exercise in the open air favors the excretion of waste matters which otherwise would be deposited in the cellular tissues. The fatty degeneration so much admired in infancy, aids in the production of emaciation and consumption at adult age.

A fat person, at whatever period of life, has not a sound tissue in his body; not only is the entire muscular system degenerated with the fatty particles,[54] but the vital organs—heart, lungs, brain, kidneys, liver, etc.—are likewise mottled throughout, like rust spots in a steel watch-spring, liable to fail at any moment.

[54] A slice of steak from the loin of a stall-fed ox exhibits this disease very clearly: mark its "well mixed" appearance (a token of praise to the ignorant or reckless epicure), where the muscular

tissue has given place to the globules of fat which denote unexcreted excess in diet, and deficient nutrition, from lack of exercise.

The gifted Gambetta, whom M. Rochefort styled a "fatted satrap," died (far under his prime) because of this depraved condition: a slight gun-shot wound, from which a "clean" man would have speedily recovered, ended this obese diabetic's life. Events sufficiently similar are constantly occurring on both sides of the water; every hour men are rolling into ditches of death because they do not learn how to live. These ditches have fictitious names—grief, fright, apoplexy, heart disease, kidney troubles, etc., etc.—but the true name is *chronic self-abuse*.

Says an agricultural journal: "The eggs of most fowls are infertile from too much pampering and too little exercise. It is not wise to fatten any animal intended for breeding purposes." The principle here involved does not relate simply to the fertility of the ovum, but to the health and stamina of all living creatures: fat is disease. Very fat women can not conceive, or, if they do, their children can not be born alive; and those who are to any degree degenerated in this manner can not endow their offspring with the full measure of vitality to which they are justly entitled; while too often they are foredoomed to sickly lives and premature deaths.

I can in no way better illustrate the relation of fat to health and strength, than by repeating the remarks of an intelligent and observing young farmer. "I fatten my cattle," said he, "because it pays—the market demands fat creatures; so I have my barn very snug and warm, and feed high. My neighbor, on the other hand, is what would be called a 'poor farmer'; that is, his buildings are not of the best, his barn has broad cracks all around, which gives them pure air, and his cattle are never fat. He works his oxen hard, gives them enough to eat to keep them in full health and vigor, but nothing for adipose. Mornings, in winter, when he turns his oxen out into the yard, they prance out like a lot of colts, kick up their heels and shake their horns like healthy creatures as they are; while mine will almost tumble down over the door-sill! His cows never give as much milk nor make as much butter as mine; but they are never sick, while mine are sometimes, and I lose one now and then with 'milk-fever,' or some other disease resulting from high feeding; but I am farming for profit, and my heifers bring an extra price by reason of the great milk and butter record of their mothers, and I can afford to have a sick or even a dead cow occasionally, providing I keep the fact quiet—not advertise the danger of the process necessary to 'drive the milk out of them.'"

[Obesity being a disease peculiar to, and (terminating in cholera infantum or some zymotic disease) especially fatal in, infancy, the author has endeavored to treat the subject exhaustively in his work entitled "How to Feed the Baby." He would merely observe, in this connection, that in plant life or animal life, the universal law is a *lean, lank infancy*: those creatures and those slips which thrive continuously and reach a healthy maturity are *never* fat or stocky during the period of growth. The human infant only is sought to be made an exception to this rule; with what success the mortality reports fully attest.]

CHAPTER VIII.

BILIOUSNESS, "HAY FEVER," NEURALGIA, ETC.

Regarding this ridiculous (because unnecessary) disorder, Sir Lionel Beale, a recognized authority, says: "The bilious 'habit' seems to be due to an unusually sensitive, irritable stomach and liver, which will discharge their functions fairly in a moderate degree, but which can not be made to do more than this without getting much out of order, [unless, I would remark, the *needs* of the system be augmented and, consequently, the digestive powers exalted, by means of increased exercise, less pampering, more outdoor air, the use of lighter clothing, etc.] Most of the organs" he goes on to say, "taking part in the digestion and assimilation of food seem to strike work when the bilious attack comes on. [It would seem more accurate to say that the 'strike,' resulting from overtaxation—excessive and unwholesome alimentation—constitutes the 'attack']. If food be taken, the suffering becomes greater. The fact seems to be, that the digestive organs require rest for a time, and if, when an attack comes on, this rest is given, the bilious state passes off, and the patient then feels extremely well, perhaps for a considerable time. Persons of the 'bilious habit' should not [who should?] eat 'rich' foods, fatty matters, fried dishes, etc., etc., and should shun alcohol." He advises little or no meat; commends the vegetarian diet, fruits, and a good proportion of whole-meal bread—corn, rye, and wheat. The free use of milk promotes biliousness, in many cases. Skim-milk often "agrees" when whole milk can not be taken in any quantity without causing much disturbance. Milk can not be called a natural food for man, and, indeed, many are obliged to relinquish its use altogether; besides, as remarked elsewhere, there is much disease among cows, owing to the unnatural manner of feeding them, and in such cases the milk is impure. It is a safe rule for bilious subjects to abstain from milk altogether; while butter, cream and cheese are still more objectionable.

In the following complaints the benefit derived from temporary abstinence from food are most marked; the acute symptoms, as catarrhal discharges, feverishness, or pain, shortly disappear (when the fast may be broken), and the disorders themselves may be eradicated by a wholesome regimen such as would, in the first instance, have prevented them: acute catarrh, "rose," or "hay" fever, influenza, feverishness, fever (one to six days, or until convalescence), neuralgia (including headache and toothache). The list might be extended somewhat, but enough has been said to illustrate the principle that "fresh air, fasting, and exercise is Nature's triple panacea" for the pain and discomfort experienced in a wide range of disorders where the necessity exists for excreting poisonous elements, and resting the viscera concerned in alimentation. "This exasperation of irritation *in the viscera*, and for the most part in the ganglionic network about the stomach and liver," says an eminent medical author, "is an invariable concomitant and cause" [of neuralgia, and all chronic nerve aches].

HINTS AND APHORISMS.

A well-knit frame never "drops a stitch."—A chilly person is a sick person: good health, not good clothes, nor artificial heat, keeps a man feeling warm.—A rear guard: "I shall bring him out of this all right," says the doctor,—"if no new complication arises"; and then he prescribes a drug or a compound of drugs, which tends to provoke the complication. For hundreds of years it has been, and, in general practice, still is the aim in sickness, to excite the organism to greater exertion in this, that or the other direction, *by giving it more to do*; the new gospel teaches that the true theory is, to enable Nature to put forth her energies in the most life-saving manner, albeit in her own fashion, by giving her more to do *with*: fresh air, sunshine, cleanliness, water,—the latter *pure, i.e.,* without the everlasting drug which constitutes the "more to do." It is a hackneyed expression, that "a man is either a fool or his own physician at forty"; but if he then find himself neither whole nor mending, he is a fool if he does not seek advice. Stomach digestion demands a period of leisure; hence the rule, "Never eat till you have leisure to digest."—Assimilation and nutrition demand peace of mind, to ensure the best results; in sickness, especially, "the balance of power" often lies in this direction.

Note.—It should be understood that aside from the above hint, the foregoing disorders are to be considered by the reader in connection with the teachings of this volume as a whole. (See concluding paragraph in the chapter on Bright's Disease.)

Having studied the subject well and with all practicable aid, settle upon a regimen, let it become second nature, and never worry about diet or think of your stomach; but if that organ persists in making itself *felt*, adopt a more abstemious regimen still, and go on again.

Maria Giberne—artist and vegetarian, of whom at the age of fifty, Mozley said: "She is the handsomest woman I ever saw," and who "now at near eighty has the same flowing locks, though they are white as snow, and her talk and her letters are as bright as ever"—ascribed her wonderful preservation and unfailing health to her observation of the fasts [she was a Catholic] and her general abstemiousness. "Her diet consisted chiefly of bread and fruit, mostly apples. One apple in the middle of a long day she spoke of as a great refreshment. She had never to complain of the heat."

We call it a disorder when Nature is really putting things to rights—bringing the order of health out of the chaos of disease: it is like "house-cleaning," where the mistress has let things run at loose ends for a long time—sweeping the dirt under the stove, behind the door, etc., and making unnecessary dirt—instead of *keeping* the establishment in order and thereby avoiding any occasion for a general upsetting.

Says one of Boston's eloquent preachers, the Rev. M. J. Savage: "In nine cases out of ten, men and women might fairly be called to account for being sick"; and Dr. T. L. Nichols, the eminent hygienist of London, says the same thing, only in slightly different language: "In nine cases out of ten, if people, when they found themselves becoming sick, would simply stop eating, they would have no need of drugs or doctors."

A certain class of temperance reformers sign pledges to be moderate in their indulgences, and not to "treat" or be "treated." This rule would be a hundred-fold more life-saving applied (rationally) to food than to drink. It is quite generally the custom to urge our friends to eat to repletion, when they partake of our hospitality.

Given a natural mode of life and natural food, the appetite also would be natural, and the stomach would not accept more than it could digest.

Nature appears, often, to be a lenient creditor, but she never neglects to collect her little bill, finally, with interest and costs of suit: "In the physical world there is no forgiveness of sin."

The mandate, In the sweat of thy face shalt thou eat bread, has, in my opinion, a physiological basis: a man can eat with advantage only an amount corresponding to the exertion he puts forth,—a modicum being allowed, of course, for the physiological labor of the organism.

"Do not think these are unimportant things [questions of diet, etc.], not dignified enough to be spoken of in the pulpit. I tell you they reach to your mind and to your morals; they reach to your theology; they reach clear to heaven, so far as you are concerned, and are of fundamental importance, touching your religious and moral life a good deal more, sometimes, than what you think about the Bible, Sunday, or any other religious institution whatever."—SAVAGE.

"Nothing hurts me—I eat everything." (Next year): "Nothing agrees with my stomach—I can't eat anything." Thus the dyspeptics' ranks are kept full with recruits from those who "don't want any advice about diet."

"Indigestion is charged by God with enforcing morality on the stomach."—THOLEMYÉS.

Every appetite held in check, aids in restraining every other—making *all* serve the man, instead of the man them; while every one let loose, tends powerfully to give free rein to all.

CHAPTER IX.

THE FLESH-FOOD FALLACY

[See Chapter III.]

demands more than the passing notice accorded to it in the chapters on Consumption: The facts of chemistry are eternal and indisputable, as are all the truths of science; but, as between two kinds of aliment, or two substances which are being considered as to their adaptation to the purpose of nourishing the body, while chemistry accurately points out which contains the greatest amount of this or that constituent, and is often of service, as affording data for a presumption, in the absence of definite knowledge, she often fails to discover—despite the chemist's, or rather his blind pupil's dogmatic assertion to the contrary—which is really the *most natural,* and consequently the *best adapted* for the purpose of alimentation. In nothing do we observe this more strikingly than in a comparison between flesh and vegetable foods. A three-column criticism of a former work (How to Feed the Baby), in one of our leading magazines, and which sums up its merits by "hoping the book will be read by all on whom devolves the important duty, the care of children; for it is an effort to institute the correct principle of feeding 'the baby,'" contains the following upon the subject of animal *vs.* vegetable food: "We discover," says the critic, "on page 98 that our author is a vegetarian, after all. In speaking of a nutritious diet whereby to enrich the breast milk, he makes the following startling statement: 'Unleavened bread, or mush, made from the unbolted meal of wheat, rye, or corn, has *very much more nutriment,* pound for pound, than is contained in beef or mutton, notwithstanding the fallacy that classes the latter as hearty food.' This is only a declaration without proof, contrary to all authority on foods. We take the following table from Prof. Johnston's 'Chemistry of Common Life':

	Lean beef.	Wheaten bread.
Water and blood	77	40
Myosin or gluten	19	7
Fat	3	1
Starch	0	50
Salt and other mineral mat.	1	2

"From which is deduced the fact, that ordinary flesh is about three times as rich in myosin or gluten as ordinary wheaten bread, or, in other words, a pound of beefsteak is as nutritious as three pounds of wheaten bread. In a second edition of Dr. Page's book, we hope he will correct this great error."

It should be stated that bread made from whole, *i.e.*, unbolted and *unsifted*, meal, is much richer in gluten and certain invaluable salts, than shown in the figures here given.

Because the most careful observation on the part of intelligent and conscientious men who have had the best opportunities for ascertaining the relative merits of these two classes of foods, viz.: nutrients proper, and the stimulo-nutrients, or, in other words, foods which are naturally adapted to the human organism, and those substances (as, for example, the flesh of animals) which, along with a great deal of nourishment, contain elements which, being of an excretory and noxious character, *excite* or *stimulate* the organism, and are, consequently, to that degree injurious—because, I would repeat, the proof is, in my estimation, overwhelmingly in favor of vegetable food, more particularly the cereals and fruits, so far from contemplating the "correction of this great error," I desire to reassert, most emphatically, as a fundamental truth in dietetics, and in no sense an error, that, pound for pound, the cereal grains are not only more nutritious (speaking of their effects upon the human organism) than flesh, but, physiologically speaking, they are free from the impurities which abound in the latter, and which are often rendered still more noxious by the presence of actual disease among animals *fattened* for human food.

The advocates of flesh-food have a marvelous faculty for misrepresenting some facts, and for the non-presentation of others which should appear if the discussion is for the purpose of deciding the question on its merits. To illustrate: I find in Johnson's Encyclopedia (Article on Hygiene, by a prominent physician) the following: "It must be admitted that men can, under favorable circumstances, exist through long periods without meat. This is shown in the instances of many tribes in Asia and Africa, who live almost entirely on rice and other grains, and also by many of the peasantry of Continental Europe, and the Scotch Highlanders who are confined to a diet containing very little animal food. Yet it is equally true that men can exist on meat alone, as is done by the Indian riders of the South American pampas, for months together." But the writer of the above (from ignorance of the fact, doubtless,) does not add, that those races who live upon a well-selected vegetable diet excel in every way—mentally, morally, and physically—those races or tribes who subsist entirely on flesh. What would the above authority call "favorable circumstances" such as would enable men to "exist" without meat? Was he thinking of the French officers, prisoners of war, who were fed, for a year or more, on rice and Indian corn exclusively, with water for their only drink, to return to their commands in improved health, to receive promotion by reason of vacancies occasioned by the death of comrades who had been favored with an abundance of meat? Or of the muscular Japanese, hard-working men and finely developed women of whom a recent sojourner in Japan says: "The quantity of food they eat is astonishingly small when compared with the food devoured by meat-eaters from the Western world.... Seemingly their frames are as tough as steel, not susceptible of cold or intense heat—going thinly clad in freezing weather, and not shrinking from the sun in its most oppressive season.... They are a marvel of strength, and illustrate the lesson that health, strength, and endurance may exist on a light and scanty diet of rice and vegetables, together with fish. The Rikisha men are not so heavily molded, being of much slighter build, but they are also full of muscle, though not so prodigally developed [as with the class of laborers before referred to]. The fatigue these men undergo and withstand can be partially estimated when it is remembered that it is not considered an extraordinary feat for them to travel forty miles a day with their seated passenger. No matter how hot it may be, while the passenger is complaining of the heat, he is being whirled along and protected by his umbrella from the rays of the sun, and the motive power never flags. This Rikisha man keeps up a pace like a deer, his body generally bare to the sun, being guiltless of clothing that could inconvenience the free movement of the body or limbs. He takes but the slightest quantity of refreshment while on the road—a cup of tea and a modicum of rice being the extent of his gormandizing during the travel. And they repeat these exploits day after day, never eating meat." Of the women this writer remarks: "With beautifully rounded arms and limbs, with smallest of feet and hands, and small-boned, they present the spectacle of what the human form should be in its natural grace and finish.... The women, young and old, are seen bearing loads upon their backs that the uninitiated in such work would not be able to stand up under. They will travel miles laden this way with a speed that would suffice to tire an average Western woman if entirely unincumbered. In fact few of our women could at all walk the distance the old women do here while bearing heavy loads. And all this is performed on an abstemious vegetable diet." Thus it would seem that "the most favorable circumstances," to use the language of Johnson's contributor, to enable men and women to live "without meat," are plenty of hard work in the open air,[55] and a somewhat restricted diet; for it must be remembered that the people of whom we have been speaking, are from necessity the least able to indulge in unlimited quantities of their peculiar food of all the people in the land.

[55] It is very generally agreed by the most eminent medical men of all schools of practice, that in the absence of free exercise in the open air, animal food *must* be abstained from.

As to the moral aspect of the question, I grant that a man can not sin without knowledge. If he believes it necessary and right for the higher animals, elevated human beings, to slaughter and feast upon the lower—the gentle, mild-eyed creatures who serve and minister unto us so patiently, so faithfully, and, indeed, so lovingly—then to kill and devour is, for him, no crime. But if men were as ready to learn from their instincts, as they are to yield to their artificial cravings, the natural loathing which all, or most people, feel at the sight of bloodshed, and which so many experience at the bare thought of taking life, would teach us the unnaturalness and therefore the harmfulness of a flesh diet. (See Appetite.)

Finally, there remains to be answered, one argument, the most rational of all that are put forward in favor of the continued use of flesh-food, viz.: heredity and habit, and a "second nature" resultant therefrom. Even some hygienic writers argue stoutly the necessity of recognizing this law, as particularly applicable to this question, and declare the absurdity of the position assumed by those who demand the abandonment of flesh-food for all who would insure to themselves the blessing of health. While affirming that the vital organism may in a few years, even, become accustomed to the *use* of almost anything, no matter how repugnant or destructive it naturally is, as opium, liquor, tobacco, etc., provided the process be gradual enough, they still hold that with regard to animal food, a substance acknowledged by them to be unwholesome, the organism can not become accustomed to its *non-use* until generations of better habits have remodeled the organism to suit the conditions. Theoretically, it would seem grossly absurd to say that when, as is the known fact, cats, dogs, bears, and the like, can thrive perfectly on a strict vegetarian diet (I have, myself, tried this successfully with the first two), that *man* alone has no hope this side the grave of being able to abandon animal food! In practice, it is found that the only thing required is to convince the mind of an individual of the unnaturalness and unwholesomeness of flesh-food; *then* if he be conscientious the battle is won, and it only remains to furnish him with a diet suited to his needs, (the selection and preparation of which, many hygienists, however, are far from comprehending fully; hence the only reason I can find for the continuance of the mixed diet in any case). But if he be either unconvinced or lacking in moral force, he can not be harmed by the presentation of the vegetarian *theory*, for he will continue his flesh-eating and take the consequences. So long, however, as any hygienist favors even a moderate indulgence in animal foods as a necessity for most people throughout their lives, his followers will take it upon themselves to decide as to what constitutes moderation, just as is the case with coffee, liquor, and tobacco-users, only the former (by reason of their ignorance as to what constitutes health and symptoms of disease) have no such means of recognizing the symptoms of excess, as have the latter. The truth is that "abstinence from *all* unwholesome practices, only, is easier than temperance."

Note.—This chapter is particularly recommended to the notice of members and friends of the American Society for the Prevention of Cruelty to Animals.

CHAPTER X.

AIR-BATHS.

With a view to the exaltation of the condition of the entire organism, as well as simply that of the digestive and assimilative system—and in addition to the reform already suggested as to clothing, *i.e.*, a reduction in the number and weight of garments habitually worn, when these have been superabundant,—I would say to all classes, sick or well, that great advantage will be derived from habituating themselves to transient exposure of the entire surface of the body to the air. Often enough, we observe persons sitting heavily clad, in a warm room and close to the fire, and yet feeling "shivery" and sure of having "caught cold." To throw off all clothing would banish such chills *instanter*, especially if the person begins to give himself a brisk hand-rubbing. The skin is sweltered, and is numb for want of circulation in the capillaries. In the case supposed the person has *prevented* a "cold." Next to the water-bath, which is, of course, or ought to be, an air-bath and water-bath combined, the simple air-bath is invaluable as a prophylactic or a curative; and in very many instances, say for several mornings in each week, and whenever the usual water-bath is not convenient, the air-bath will prove an excellent substitute. In place of *dodging* from the sweltering bed into his heavy day-clothing, the *robust* man will be far more likely to maintain his vigorous condition by doffing his night-shirt and indulging for the space of, say, five minutes or less, in brisk hand-rubbing all over, however cold his sleeping-room, and again on going to bed; while the delicate ones should, with due caution, inaugurate the same system (some *will-power* has to be exerted), but graduated, as to temperature and duration, to their special conditions—advancing as their physical condition improves under its influence until they are no longer members of that immense army—the victims of "aërophobia." Patients themselves too weak for even the exercise of self-rubbing will still derive great benefit from the air-bath, in a temperature, say, of 65°, with an attendant to rub them briskly from neck to heels. Set in practice in a rational manner this custom will never injure the most delicate person, but on the contrary will always prove beneficial. It will not bring the dead to life, nor, indeed, "cure" the moribund; but it is one of Nature's most efficient aids—it is Nature herself, in very truth—and I have seen patients who were thought to be hopelessly ill, begin to take on what seemed to be renewed life, largely through this new use of fresh air, and the *dismissal* of the *unnatural dread of it*. For example:

CHRONIC DYSPEPSIA CURED BY FASTING AND FRESH AIR.

A patient, Mrs. T., of New Hampshire, a very bright lady indeed, and one who appreciated the necessity of fresh air, had yet, through a very deep decline, in addition to a life-long invalidism, become hyper-sensitive to cold, wrapping and over-wrapping to guard against chilliness, fearful of the least current of air. Both relatives and friends were discouraged as to her recovery—it even being urged, after I had taken the case, that if, as it seemed, there were no hopes of her getting well, she ought to have some "medicine to ease her pathway to the grave."[56] This was in the month of October of the year 1882, when she came under my care. I induced her to leave off eating, since eating was particularly disagreeable, and only served to keep up the chronic inflammation of the entire digestive and neighboring viscera, causing her a great deal of suffering and threatening her with starvation. [Referring to her first letter (written by her sister), describing her condition, I find such expressions as these: "My physician, who feared heart disease, as my mother and one sister had died of it, becoming alarmed at my symptoms, desired a consultation, and Dr. ——, Professor of Cardiac

Diseases at —— —— College Hospital, was called. He said heart was all right, but lungs weak. I was well drugged, but when they stuffed me on cod-liver oil and beefsteak I would have inflammation of the stomach and liver and, of course, grew worse, with such a terrible ache at the base of my brain.... Was brought to N. H. (from Brooklyn, N. Y.) in May, and had congestion of the liver shortly after. My physician, here, ordered iron and strychnine, but it did no permanent good. All my friends say I am starving to death, and unless you can advise me, I fear that I shall, for I am terribly emaciated even now.... My æsophagus, stomach, and liver are in an irritated condition,... am sore all over,—can not sleep at night; have taken chloral by physician's advice. My flesh has a yellow-purple color—arms and hands grow quite purple at times," etc., etc.] I directed her to throw away her medicine—iron and strychnia, aconite and chloral—*bottles and all*,—as the first step, telling her that whether she was to live or die, she should be made more comfortable without, than with medicine. For the exhausted digestive organs, I directed entire rest, as before stated; and for seven days she swallowed nothing but *cool* or *hot* water.[57] *For the first three or four days many of her symptoms increased in severity*—not a bad sign. At the same time I succeeded in removing from her mind the dread of air-currents, improving the ventilation of both the sleeping and sitting room, and she, furthermore, begun the system of air-bathing here enjoined. On the seventh day she reported by letter that she felt as though something "more nourishing than water would be very acceptable," that she had some very nice pears and Delaware grapes, and would like to try them. I directed her to take a breakfast of fruit every morning; and, at night, a dinner of two or three unleavened gems (made from *unsifted* wheat-meal and mixed stiff with cold water), with a very little fruit, and a cupful of skimmed milk (no butter, cream, or any kind of animal fat), beginning with a single gem; the milk to be taken last, by itself, and each swallow to be held for a moment in the mouth. Under this treatment she is making excellent progress—not rapid and fictitious, as we often enough witness under a stimulating regimen, but a real, natural growth healthward. She rides out in all weathers, walks a mile or two every day to and from the neighbors, aids in the work about the house, and on December 9th, about two months after she began the "natural cure," she reports by postal as follows: "I am still on the hygienic tack and growing stronger, though I still have some aches to assure me that I am mortal. I 'sleep beautifully,' with window open in all weathers. I enjoy my air-baths every morning in the hall (a portion of the time), with the mercury at zero!" (She is now in robust health.)

[56] Her disease was chronic dyspepsia: the stomach was so irritable that it could seldom retain anything—at least a portion of even the smallest ordinary ration would be ejected—the liver was very much congested and enlarged; the bowels were obstinately constipated; there was extreme emaciation, and but little strength, though, generally, great good nature and cheerfulness in spite of her ailments. Had been taking chloral for wakefulness, and iron and strychnine as a tonic. She took no medicine after becoming my patient.

[57] See note 3 in Appendix, p. 279.

Benjamin Franklin had observed the invigorating effects of this practice and would often, in moderate weather, rise from bed in the morning and, entirely nude, write for an hour or more, and then dress for breakfast. When wakeful at night, the great philosopher found that by throwing off the bed-coverings for a few minutes he could then re-cover and fall asleep and sleep soundly.[58] Finally, so deeply was Franklin impressed from his own experience and observation in this direction that he proposed to cure all diseases by means of the air-bath, combined with plain and abstemious living. His idea concerning the most popular of all disorders may be inferred from the following: "I shall not attempt to explain why 'damp clothes' occasion colds rather than wet ones, because I doubt the fact. I imagine that neither the one nor the other contributes to this effect, and that the causes of colds are totally independent of wet and even of cold." (Essays, p. 216.)

[58] One may be partially stifled and made wakeful by confined air about the skin, as well as asphyxiated with bad air in the lungs. The eminent Dr. B. W. Richardson, of London, lays great stress upon the necessity, and has himself devised a means, of ventilating the space about the person in bed —a very gradual change of the air being insured. Next to any special mechanical device for the accomplishment of this object, and perhaps all sufficient generally, comes the use of loosely woven sheets and blankets, instead of heavy linen or cotton sheets and "comfortables" which are well-nigh airtight.

Dr. James R. Nichols, of Boston, the well-known scientist, thus emphasizes the importance of this form of bath:

"One of the most sagacious, far-seeing men this country has produced was Doctor Franklin. He was in all that he did and said far in advance of his age and of his opportunities, and his wisdom was of that rare kind which does not grow old. His discoveries and devices were not partial and imperfect, but such as have needed little revision or improvement.

"The lightning-rod he devised is to-day the best form we have, and his method of applying it to buildings needs no special modification. His open-fireplace stove is still largely in use, no better one having been devised. His philosophical theories and speculations were so rounded out, so clearly and sagaciously developed, that many of them stand to-day as fixed facts in philosophy and science. Among his important discoveries was the 'air-bath,' a sanitary or curative agent which is of the highest consequence to the welfare of mankind. It may be said that he did not present the matter in much practical detail, but he suggested it, used it, and gave reasons for believing in its high importance.

"We have made the air-bath a matter of careful study, and wish to call the attention of the readers of the *Journal* to it, as a means of securing and preserving health, which is of the first importance. It is impossible for physicians or individuals of ordinary sagacity to fail to see that a large proportion of invalids and semi-invalids do not bear well the application of either cold or tepid water to the body. A man or woman must naturally be of strong constitution and in robust health to arise in the morning, in cold climates, and stand under the icy streams which come from a shower-bath, without breaking down in health at an early day. The sponge-bath is less injurious, but it saps the vitality of many to a fatal extent, and feeble persons are rarely in any degree benefited by its use. The tepid bath, as a curative means, constantly followed weakens rather than strengthens, and many can not continue it for the space even of a week. Bathing, beyond the needs of perfect cleanliness, is not generally to be recommended. Mankind are not aquatic animals, like ducks and geese; they are not born on or in the water, and nature never designed that they should be splashing about in that element within the lines of the temperate or frigid zones....

"The air-bath is a means of recuperation which needs to be intelligently and carefully adopted, and like all other good things must not be abused. There are hundreds of thousands of people of both sexes, in this country, who lead miserable lives, and yet they are not in bed, not perhaps confined to their dwellings; they suffer from nervous prostration, from imperfect digestion and assimilation, from worry, from overwork, from the care of households, etc. A vast number in the mighty army of invalids are not themselves to blame for their physical weaknesses; their idiosyncrasies of organization come by inheritance....

"Now, the air-bath comes to the feeble and physically impoverished as a kind and good friend; and let us see how we can obtain from it the highest good. Nearly all semi-invalids are inclined to sedentary habits, and as the circulation is languid the body in winter is under a persistent chill. In the morning, upon getting out of bed, the clothing can not be too quickly adjusted, as the body is in a shiver; and the air of a cool room is a thing to be dreaded.

"The morning is the time for the air-bath, and all that is required is a hair-cloth mitten [a towel, or even the bare hand alone will answer, however,] and a moderately cool room. When the invalid steps from the bed to the floor in the morning, let the hair glove or mitten be seized, and without removing the night-clothes proceed to rub gently all parts of the body, at the same time walking about in the room until a feeling of fatigue is experienced; then drop the glove, and gently pass the hand over all parts of the body before resuming the clothing. [Unless the nude body is extremely sensitive to cold, it may be exposed to the air for a few moments, even on the first morning]. The next morning jump out of bed in a moderately cool [never a 'close,' but always a ventilated] room, and go over the same process as before, remaining a little longer exposed to the air after the rubbing. The third morning repeat this treatment; and on the fourth, or at the end of a week, take off all the night-clothing, and briskly apply the hair glove, first with the right hand and then with the left, all the time walking about. Follow up this, as the degree of strength permits, morning after morning, until the body is so rejuvenated and the blood so attracted to the surface, that the cool air is felt to be a luxury. Let the body be entirely nude, no socks upon the feet, no scarf about the chest. At first, or after the first week, perhaps, the exposure to the pure cool air may be three or four minutes; soon increase the exposure, until, after a month or two, the air-bath may continue for twenty minutes or half an hour. Do not fail to walk about during the first month, using the hands in polishing the skin. After the first month the patient may sit in the air of the room part of the time, but constant, gentle exercise is best.

"Now, another most important curative agent connected with the air-bath is *sunlight*. In summer, sunlight is accessible, but in winter only the late risers can secure its benefits. [There is no reason why morning should be regarded as the only appropriate time for this skin-airing. On the contrary, some will find midday even better, though morning is for most persons the most convenient time. Many can not devote any other hour to this work; others will not have the energy, *i. e.*, the good sense to disrobe for an air or sun bath during the day.] If possible, sit and walk in the sunlight during the bath. It is astonishing what the direct actinic rays of the morning sun can do for an invalid, when the whole nude body is brought under its influence."

SCROFULA.

A sick niece of the Mrs. T. whose case is reported on p. 168, living in New York, learning of her aunt's "miraculous cure," resolved to renounce medication and come home for hygienic treatment. Her disease is scrofula, and her condition was such that her friends had well-nigh abandoned all hope of her recovery. With non-healing ulcers, increasing in number on body and limbs; weak, languid, with neither strength nor ambition to move about; emaciated from 120 to 88 pounds—it did seem as though her case was a most critical one, indeed. Nevertheless, on the clean, pure, nutritious diet which had restored her relative—largely "natural," wholly abstemious, and free from all animal fats (see foot-note, page 232)—modified to suit her particular needs—taken morning and night with appropriate air and water baths, etc., she soon began to show signs of improvement. After two months' trial, her aunt writes that her niece is certainly gaining. This gain must be real instead of fictitious, since it is impossible to attribute it to any artificial stimulation. The sores are beginning to heal; her strength is increasing, by exerting it daily—drawing, at first moderately, but increasing her drafts from day to day, upon the "reserved force," each draft being overpaid, so to say, by subsequent rest, food, sleep, etc., thus daily increasing her physical bank account,—there now seems every prospect that this young wife will ere long be restored to her home as good as new. [Both aunt and niece take their meals in their private rooms, alone, the total quantity and variety to be taken at each meal only appearing on the table; there is, therefore, no temptation for "trying a little more" of this, that, and the other thing, which almost inevitably leads to excess, and consequent impairment of appetite; no taxing of the sick brain to be "agreeable" to a "tableful" of healthy persons, to interfere with the digestion.]

CHAPTER XI.

SALINE STARVATION—CAUTION.

The danger to which I am about to allude—a real danger, as I believe—does not refer to abstinence from artificial salt, but rather to the loss of certain essential elements contained in the grains, fruits, and vegetables, owing (1) to their being cooked at all, and (2) to bad cooking. Vegetables form a large proportion of the food of even those who live on the "mixed diet"; and unless cooked (see Natural Diet) in the best manner, a large part of certain of their elements may be lost, and a degree of starvation result therefrom. For example: potatoes, when peeled and over-boiled, lose nearly one-half of their potash. So, too, when they are kept boiling until the skins break open—the "mealy" potato, often preferred,—more especially if they are permitted to remain in the water any length of time thereafter, a large additional percentage of valuable matters must be dissolved and turned away with the water. The chief aim should be to retain all the elements contained in the food articles, whether the cereals, vegetables, or fruits. Hence all of those substances that are acceptable in a raw state should be thus eaten; and when any of them are cooked, it should be (referring particularly to vegetables) done upon the principle adopted by well-informed cooks in boiling meat; they put the meat into *boiling* water, let it boil vigorously for a sufficient length of time (say ten or fifteen minutes) to "close the pores," as they say, and confine the juices within the meat, and then the kettle is set back where the water will keep hot, just "simmering," until the work is completed (four to eight hours, according to size of the piece of meat). The same plan should be used in cooking vegetables, except as to time—they are "done" when the fork passes through them easily. The impoverishment of vegetables, as sometimes cooked, is poorly compensated for—not at all, in fact, except in flavor—by the use of artificial salt; while this substance, so universally used, is altogether unnatural and injurious, in proportion to the amount swallowed. The loss of the natural salines, in the manner referred to, is especially observed by vegetarians who dine at ordinary tables, where exclusion of animal food and white bread is the only selection they can make. It is of vital importance for food-reformers to understand and guard against this danger—not that they will suffer more than those who take the mixed diet, for in fact the reverse is true (their whole-meal bread being a great aid)—but being, as it were, on exhibition before the world, it is important for them to obtain and enjoy all the advantages pertaining to the system they advocate.

Says Dr. Hunter:

"It is an old and a cruel experiment, that of the French academicians, who fed dogs on washed flesh-meat until they died of starvation. The poor animals soon became aware that it was not food, and refused to eat it. Were our instincts as natural, no charming of the eyes or tickling of the palate by our cook would persuade us to swallow those washed and whitened foods that deceive us into weakness.

"Analysis of the liver and other important vital organs after death, show that in some diseased states these organs contain only one-half of certain saline matters that are invariable in the healthy organ. And not only so, but that in proportion to this deficiency the organ is useless for its work. In fact, as the organ changed its tissue (as does every part of the body every three or four years), and was compelled to renew itself in the absence of sufficient potash and phosphates, it did its best to preserve its form and structure much as a fossil does. It rebuilt itself as best it could of such material as would make tissue with the minimum of potash; but such tissue, whilst useful and conservative in retaining the form, elasticity and contractility of the organ, is as useless for secretion and excretion as a fossil liver."

The want of knowledge, not only on the part of the laity, but medical men as well, regarding such questions, and health matters in general, is exhibited in the utterances heard on every hand: "The doctor says the trouble is with my liver," explains one who hasn't a sound tissue in his entire body. "My blood is bad—so the doctor says."[59] "'He' gave me something for my blood"—or my appetite, or my kidneys as the case may be—it might as well be *for my grandmother*." "The first thing to be done," says an eminent physician, after citing an hypothetical case, "is to clear out the liver"; and then, after apologizing for "what might seem to be an unscientific expression," he continues: "I have already explained the way in which certain purgatives may be said to have the effect of clearing out the liver, and first among these we must reckon *mercurials*." The italics are my own. He then offers a generous dose of blue-pill "every night, or two or three grains of calomel either alone or combined with extract of hyoscyamos or conium, and this," he continues, "should be followed next morning by a saline draught." Mercury, to poison and exasperate the entire organism, and then a saline potion in the hope of getting rid of the mercury! And then he offers a grain of sense—a homœopathic dose, indeed, but drowned in a deluge of something vastly worse than sugar and water: "But even with all this care in food and drink, with all this attention to what is to be taken and what avoided, how are we to keep the liver in order *without exercise*?" Again, the underlining is the author's. How, indeed, without attention to all the simple laws of life—"so simple," says Schopenhauer, "that we refuse to understand them!"

[59] Strangely enough the belief prevails, generally, that the blood is a fixed quantity; whereas, in fact, it is constantly changing, second by second, used up and cast out, and replaced from the food; so that if one's blood is impure to-day, he may at once begin to make a better article, by making it of better material,—not by "tinkering it up" with drugs or so-called "blood-purifiers."

Dr. Hunter continues:

"Not only the liver, but the kidney, spleen, and brain, and the small blood-vessels in every part of the body share in this degeneration of tissue; and strangely enough (and not unlike the French experiment), this amyloid, waxy, or lardaceous tissue is indigestible by the gastric juice. It is *washed flesh* made inside the body, and is good for nothing either dead or alive.

"The washed flesh fed to those poor dogs contained abundance of nitrogen and carbon; but these alone, as Liebig remarked, were as useless as stones in the absence of saline matters—*not of common salt, be it remembered, for that is found in excess in the fossil organs mentioned*. The essential salines that can be readily washed out of food are chiefly two—potash salts and alkaline phosphates. These are also the two that are found deficient, about 50 per cent. in the waxy form of degenerated tissue. This is the type most common in atrophied children, and in persons suffering from consumption[60] and other wasting diseases; but it is not uncommon in the capillaries and small arteries of many who *seem* in health.

[60] See chapters on "Consumption."

"When vegetables are soaked in cold water to keep them fresh, when they are blanched in hot water to please our eye, or when they are well boiled and their essence drained off that we may eat the depleted residue, those soluble salines are almost entirely extracted. And what are left? Chiefly the less soluble salts of lime and magnesia—just those elements so abundant in the cretaceous degeneration of blood-vessels.

"Potash is the alkaline element of formed tissue; its absence is one great cause of scurvy, as well as of the waxy and perhaps the cretaceous types of degeneration.[61] A little examination of our modern commoner foods will show how deficient they are in this element.

[61] See chapter on "Bright's Disease."

"Bread was, I suppose, at one time, the 'staff of life,' but it could hardly have been white bread. Of it, one pound contains about seven grains of potash, or nearly twenty grains less than a pound of brown bread. Potatoes, if peeled, steeped and boiled in plenty of water, contain only about twenty-one grains in the pound, as against thirty-seven if boiled in their skins. The skins surpass the center about four-fold in salines. Cabbages and all leafy vegetables lose much more, as the water gets right through every portion of them.

"Arrowroot, cornflour, and most of those prepared foods are more deceitful than the washed flesh of the French academicians. Stewed fruits, as made by some cooks, are also guilty of the wash. Even porridge, haricot beans, pease, etc., are by some cooks soaked when raw (this water being thrown away), and thus much depleted." After simple washing, all vegetables, including beans and pease, if soaked at all, should be boiled in the water in which they are soaked; and, finally, the water from which the cooked vegetables are withdrawn, should be used as "soup stock" thickened with bread, rice, or sliced vegetables, and seasoned with meat, if meat is used at all. Containing as it does a large percentage of the salts from the vegetables, this water supplies the necessary "seasoning" far better than artificial salt. Turnips, instead of being sliced before boiling, should be boiled whole. Onions are every way better boiled before peeling. At first, the taste, accustomed to the flavor (!) of depleted vegetables,—or rather to the condiments with which they are prepared, has to be educated to the real flavor of *whole* food. And, again, such food being more nutritious, less in amount must be eaten, upon pain of indigestion. "No wonder if this generation finds itself degenerating. Like a ship built of rotten timber, a man fed on depleted food goes all very well in good weather and with a light load; but when one can neither bear an average load, nor undergo unusual fatigue, let him cross-question his cook."[62]

[62] Charles D. Hunter, M.D., F.C.S., in *Herald of Health*.

The truth is that, to a very great degree, we build our bodies out of blood made from impure materials: (1) in part from food depleted by cooking or improper cooking, (2) in part from substances which, as all are agreed, can be "indulged in" only to a limited extent (who can define the limit?), (3) in great measure, from fermented, instead of well-digested food; —and having thus built up "fossil" bodies (still more fossilized by the use of unnatural drinks which "prevent the waste of tissue"), there must be sickness. There is no escape from it, except by a "right about face." The zymotic, and the various acute diseases, so called, are in point of fact acute *remedies* for chronic *disease*.

CHAPTER XII.

WHEAT-MEAL VS. "ENTIRE FLOUR."

Without doubt, certain brands of "whole-wheat flour," so called, are a great improvement over the article in universal demand among poor and rich alike, the white flour of commerce, in this: they are, when made by honest manufacturers, less impoverished than the white flours. In public and in private, I have advised their use instead of white flour, but solely upon the ground that the wheat is *less* robbed of certain of its invaluable constituents in the former; but I can not conceive it possible to separate the hull from the kernel without real loss, even if the hull were, in itself, objectionable, which, so far from being true, is, in my opinion, a mistake and a very serious one. The theory upon which the objection to the outside coat of the grain rests, is that this coat is composed of woody fiber, entirely indigestible and devoid of nutritive matters, and, worst of all, say these honest objectors, the hulls are coarse, sharp-edged, and irritating to the stomach and intestines, and therefore injurious in their action, especially in the case of "sensitive and delicately organized individuals." I will not stop to discuss the question as to the propriety of the phrase *sensitive and delicately organized*, as applied to the class of poor, suffering wretches who by reason of their gross habits—and I mean simply the dietetic habits of the people, not the mechanic, the artisan, the small trader, nor yet the factory hand, nor the wretched poor, but the *human race*, from the kings, queens, and presidents all along the line—who by reason, I repeat, of the universal system of diet, have become dyspeptic. I can not, however, forbear the remark, that the most sensitive and delicately organized individuals, among the most noble of all animals next to man,—and in some aspects far superior to him,—the horse, in his finest and most delicate state, finds a perfect food in the whole grain, chewing it himself. I may be, in the minds of some, weakening my argument by comparing the digestive apparatus of man with that of the horse, but I am desirous of impressing upon the minds of my readers the well-known but imperfectly considered fact, that our horse-fanciers,—who dote on their hundred-thousand-dollar animals, and who would place before them the most costly and complicated dishes, certainly would feed them on the finest and whitest of flour,—"Imperial Granum" even, at drug-store prices, if it were desirable, or even not pernicious in a health point of view,—really keep their dearest pets on *bread and water*; and that, because of this, and the absence of all the hot, stimulating articles, solid or fluid, indulged in by their owners, and their regular and moderate diet of *uncooked* food, and their superior hygiene in certain essential matters, our thorough-bred horses are generally saved from becoming fat, sick, mean, wheezy, or dyspeptic, like their masters and mistresses, men, women, and children.

We know that the microscope shows up the ragged edges of the hulls and gives them a fearful aspect; but if the microscope could reason, and if it was given to arguing all questions submitted to it, I fancy it would speedily silence these objections to wheat-meal, so far as they rest upon the matter of the coarseness and the irritating capacity of the hull, by asking the microscopist to take a little glance at the stomach itself: an internal view of the digestive tract would disclose the fact that, even in the case of the most "sensitive and finely organized" subject, the lining of the stomach, for example, bears a stronger resemblance to a *quartz mill* than do these terrible hulls to sticks and stones. The trouble has been with those who seek to improve too much over Nature's methods, and especially is this the case in the question under discussion, they have reasoned mainly from one side of the question. Machinery has accomplished no end of good things, and without doubt has even greater victories yet in store, in its legitimate field; but that field is not in the line of improving on the food that Nature provides for us humans. It can and does improve over the old methods of sowing, reaping, threshing, and cleansing the various grains—no one desires to dispute this; but when the ripe, clean kernel of wheat, for instance, is placed before us, the office of machinery is ended, except so far as crushing the grain for those whose teeth or temper will not admit of chewing it. A shrewd though illiterate stable keeper said to me, in advocating whole, instead of cracked corn for horses and cattle, "it gets the juice of their teeth, and does them twice as much good. Give them meal, or cracked corn, and they don't have to chew it long enough to get the right action of the saliva."

People who neglect the most obvious hygienic rules, thereby bringing upon themselves sickness and pain, and search for special articles of diet that may seem to promise relief, remind me of a junk-dealer who would pass by old stoves, pots, kettles, and crowbars, and search for a needle in a hay-stack! The theory of the anti-wheat-meal men seems plausible at first sight, and it has been held, temporarily, by some very sound men; but one after another these have dropped it as untenable. To be sure, the ranks are kept full by new recruits, who join faster than the *thinkers* fall out. There are a thousand dyspeptics for every discerning man, and, in any event, all such—all persons, in fact, are to be congratulated when they adopt a compromise in the shape of fine flour which claims to give them all the essential elements of the wheat, and yet save their "delicate" and sensitive stomachs needless labor and irritation. But I find that the class who are *saving lives* constantly, hold to the entire meal as the only means of securing perfect bread—the staff of life.

Says Oswald: "We can not breathe pure oxygen. For analogous reasons bran flour [whole meal] makes better bread than bolted flour; meat and saccharine fruits are healthier than meat extracts and pure glucose. In short, artificial extracts and compounds are, on the whole, less wholesome than the palatable products of nature. In the case of bran-flour and certain fruits with a large percentage of wholly innutritious matter, chemistry fails to account for this fact, but biology suggests the mediate cause: the normal type of our physical constitution dates from a period when the digestive organs of our (frugivorous) ancestors adapted themselves to such food—a period compared with whose duration the age of grist-mills and made dishes is but of yesterday."

This doctoring of the cereals can never prove of service in the end, except to the manufacturers and dealers; these "preparations," however honestly made, and supposing for argument's sake that the machinery accomplishes what the manufacturers intend, will never, in and of themselves,—*i. e.*, except so far as they take the place of *white flour*—prove beneficial to mankind, and least of all to sick people, valetudinarians, and the sedentary classes,—the very ones who need the best. Imagine a constipated dyspeptic, with a heavy fur coat on his tongue, and, of course, a heavier one on the lining of his stomach—his entire alimentary canal so covered with this morbid growth that digestion and absorption are well-nigh prohibited—alarmed lest the microscopic particles of wheat-hulls should injure his delicate and sensitive inwards! "Delicate!" "sensitive!" why, it takes half a cupful of salts to move them, and that but faintly, while a pint of strong coffee makes no impression; when if they were even normally sensitive a tablespoonful of the former, or a single cup of the latter, would purge them violently. Sensitive! they are *dead*, or at least dying. Why, for this class of patients, I would sooner *add the straw* than remove the hull, as better calculated, by all odds, to meet the necessities of their condition. On the other hand, when the disease assumes the opposite form—when the tongue is raw, and the intestinal tract acutely inflamed, and from any cause preternaturally sensitive—there is but one thing in the Materia Medica of Nature that is absolutely fit to swallow, and that is *pure water*. (See Chronic Dyspepsia.) It matters not what else is comforting, temporarily,—medicine, gruel, beef-tea, milk, or what not,—the comfort and advantage are derived solely from the water, which constitutes three-fourths to nine-tenths of the whole; the other elements being injurious, and, often enough, fatal, preventing as they do the healing of the inflamed mucous membrane.

CHAPTER XIII.

FRUIT.

It is with difficulty that one who comprehends the question can restrain his impatience when people talk about the danger of indulging in fruit in summer or at any other season. "Better leave an order on the doctor's slate," says the would-be wit, when his friend passes with a watermelon or some early apples or peaches. As spring and summer come along, fruit is altogether natural, even if it does come from a little further South. That is one of the advantages of having railroads. These unwise people who dare not eat fruit, or eat it sparingly, while they stick to their winter diet of meat, grease, pastry, coffee, etc., are the ones who have the cholera morbus and other equally ridiculous things. It sometimes happens that these good people have had a "scare" in this fashion: one eats an excessive meal of fat and lean meats, old vegetables, with *plenty of gravy*, etc., all hot and heating, and calculated to create a febrile condition of the system, and insure an "attack" of indigestion. He has also eaten a piece of watermelon or other fruit—the only pure, natural substance appropriate for the time he has swallowed for the day. If, under these circumstances, he is routed at midnight, he declares he will never eat another piece of melon as long as he lives! It may be that the fruit, if he ate liberally of it, was the exciting cause of the *clearing out* that otherwise might not have taken place just then; if so, he should congratulate himself that he has been saved a later attack that might have cost him his life. Had he eaten double the quantity of fruit on an *empty stomach*, providing his system was in decent condition, there would have been no startling consequences. The stomach which refuses to accept raw fruit, or with which it does not "agree," is like that of the drunkard which rebels against pure water. When anyone has become diseased to that degree the sooner he begins to reform his habits the better. In 1863 I was captured by the Confederates and marched out of Brazier City, La., and taken to Shreveport. When captured, I had diarrhœa—the result of a flesh-food diet, wine, and all the "good things of life." The disease became chronic, and I was near dying. The melon season was on (it was in July), and in sheer desperation, ignorant of the benefits to result from it, rather expecting disaster, I ate freely of watermelon. For eight or ten days I took no other food or drink, but with this I filled myself twice a day, and a return to perfect health was the result; all trace of bowel trouble had disappeared. I have since had many opportunities for observing the benefit arising from the use of watermelon and *nothing else*, in diarrhœa, upon various persons, young and old, and I have never observed any harmful results from its use; though it is often made the scapegoat, as indicated above.

In a certain little borough in a neighboring State there was little or no fruit, not even apples, to any amount. There was a great deal of sickness every summer—diarrhœa, dysentery, fevers, etc. One enterprising resident planted an orchard—a generous one in size—and its owner was generous also. He didn't watch the neighbors' children very closely—not as closely as he did his own—and true to boys' instincts they hooked apples, green apples, little bits of apples, hard and sour, and they ate them freely. The children of the owner of that orchard did not eat green apples, for their father, although believing in fruit, thought it must be ripe to be "healthy." His children had the regularly recurring summer complaints, but the little apple-stealers did not. Without doubt fruit is more truly wholesome ripe than green; and I would here remark, that the craving for vegetable acids which these boys had, and which most children experience, would not be felt if they were properly fed at home. Still, one may eat too much even of fruit: "gold in the morning, silver at noon, and lead at night," might better be changed to diamonds, gold, and silver; and but for other considerations, unappreciated by those who fancy that it is "heavy" at eve, there would be a restriction in almost anything at the last meal sooner than in fruit. Careful observers have remarked that fruit is a prophylactic, and is also curative, taken on an empty stomach, but is likely to promote indigestion if added to a hearty meal of mixed food.[63] This is one way of saying: after having already over-eaten, or having eaten enough, eat nothing more. Surely any kind of fruit added would be less injurious than to swallow another plate of the soup, fish, or meat. The old Roman gluttons used to take an emetic after dinner; and in this country it has been the custom in times past with some, and it is not altogether obsolete even now, to take a "dinner-pill" before or after the principal meal. The morning draught of "seltzer" or other laxative, so common at the present day, serves the same purpose; and those people who, after obstinate constipation, feel comparatively happy over a violent purging from some form of artificial physic, are the ones who warn against using much fruit, because, upon some occasion, it may have performed a similar service, though without any of the injurious effects of the drugs. In warm weather the diet may well consist largely of fruit and succulent vegetables. Scrofulous children, especially, might live solely on fruit for days together, with great advantage. Such children should live in the open air as much as possible, and their sleeping-rooms should have the most thorough ventilation. If their noses and ears run in consequence of "exposure," never forget that these poisonous matters are better out than in, and that whatever aids in their elimination is curative. A simpler and purer diet will prevent the formation of catarrhal or scrofulous matters. Any degree of restriction in the matter of air and exercise can only be counteracted by a corresponding restriction in diet; but a generous allowance of all three is the safest rule. Sedentary persons, loiterers at the mountains or by the sea, can not easily make the proportion of fruit too large, even if during a torrid wave they eat little else. It should be taken at the regular meal hour only, to insure the greatest degree of health and comfort, should be thoroughly masticated, and the quantity may be just short of causing pressure at the kidneys, or flatulency, yet enough to prevent thirst. Three meals might then be indulged in with safety. The heavy dishes —meats, gravies, greasy articles, hot condiments, pastry, hot stimulating drinks—things that even in winter, in this climate, are only tolerated, and that but poorly, are deadly now, as the mortality reports, and lists of those who are said to have succumbed to the heat, attest. Moreover, for every one who pays the penalty with his life, tens of thousands are lying or sitting about, suffering the tortures of the damned, often; and all for a few minutes extra palate-tickling, or unnatural indulgences, rather,—for, leaving out the really unseasonable articles and condiments, they might revel in ripe fruits with comparative impunity. He is a poor student in dietetics, a thoughtless observer, even, who can not so regulate his eating as to regard summer as the most agreeable season of the year,—the most comfortable,—who can not bid defiance to the heated term and laugh at the danger of "sunstroke" though running a foot-race under the noonday sun. Calorific food, superadded to the predisposition already existing, is the real source of these strokes in every instance, the external heat furnishing, to be sure, the "last straw."

[63] As before intimated, only the stomach disordered and enervated from the use of hot and stimulating kinds of solid and liquid food, spices and condiments, refuses to "agree" with pure, ripe fruits. Such a stomach requires a fast day, followed by the plainest and most abstemious diet, with a gradually increasing proportion of fruit as the stomach recovers "tone." In all cases fruit requires to be thoroughly masticated, and reduced as nearly as possible to a fluid state before being swallowed.

CHAPTER XIV.

THE ONE-MEAL SYSTEM.

In this note I propose to do little more than record a few instances, out of many, of persons who have lived for longer or shorter periods, and continue to live, on one meal a day, and let my readers draw their own inferences, merely remarking that these cases have a very great significance as bearing upon the question of the *quantity of food* best suited to nourish the body and promote health. Dr. Abernethy, a celebrated English physician, affirmed that "one-fourth of all a man eats sustains him; the balance he retains at his risk"; but his countrymen eat four meals, at least.

The case of Mrs. Solberg, an emaciated dyspeptic, whose restoration to health was accomplished by the one-meal vegetarian diet and "a change of air" (at home), is mentioned in the chapter on Malaria.

S. N. Silver,[64] of Auburn, Me., a hard-working mechanic, has, for upwards of three years, lived on the one-meal-a-day plan. He eats at night, after resting sufficiently from his day's work. He never eats more than seven meals per week, not even so much as an apple between meals; and on Sundays, unless he takes considerable exercise, his "meal" consists of fruit only—three or four apples, for example. He is a typically healthy young man, and has not in three years experienced a moment of physical inconvenience. He is a vegetarian, and lives wholly on simple, pure food, chiefly bread and fruit.

[64] Mr. Silver is 30 years old and is 6 feet, 2 inches in height. On the three-meal system his greatest weight was 137 pounds. For two years past, on the new plan, he has weighed from 150 to 160 pounds, according to his work. When he works hard he eats more, and gains in weight; when his

work is light he eats light and his weight falls off correspondingly. This illustrates a truly physiological diet. It should always be thus with man and the domestic animals alike. In practice, however, the reverse is the rule: the weight increases during leisure and decreases when hard work is done. Both our athletes and race-horses are permitted to fatten between times, and are fitted for sharp work by reducing their weight by exercise. In other words, they are allowed to become diseased, and then they are "cured." This process is apt to result, finally, in premature death, or at least so exhausts the vital forces as to render former accomplishments impossible, at an age when the individual should be in his prime.

Mrs. Wieman, a sister of the above, has, for upwards of a year, taken but one meal a day, although she prepares three hot meals for her husband and several boarders. She does the entire household work for her family, which during the past summer consisted of nine adults. Her one meal (taken at noon because the regular dinner is at that hour and furnishes a better variety) is no more in amount than her dinner formerly, when she took breakfast and supper in addition. She is a perfect specimen of robust health, and finds that she can now perform with ease an amount of labor which formerly would have been a severe tax, even if possible to accomplish. Her diet is mainly vegetarian; she eats but little meat, and that only because it is constantly before her; and she avoids white flour and most forms of pastry altogether, as well as hot stimulating drinks, condiments, spices, etc., although her table is bountifully supplied with all such things.

Still another of this family, a busy milliner, has lived in this manner for several months, and finds herself improved in health by the means.

Aside from the immense amount of knowledge gained through vivisection—through dead animals, I may say—the *lives* of the lower animals teach us what to do, in some respects, as well as what to avoid. Alas, for humanity—claiming such superiority—in both classes there are important lessons which are not generally learned and practiced. As bearing upon the one-meal system, I will let Capt. B., an old hunter, tell his experience with his fox-hound: "The old fellow," said the Captain, "knows when I am going on a tramp as well as my wife does—when I turn out for a hunt, in the morning—and he won't touch a mouthful of food.[65] I used to try and 'fool' him, by acting as if I wasn't going out at all, and sometimes I could get him to eat breakfast. But I never try that game now, for I noticed, after a while, that when he fixed himself, he did better work than when I managed to get a breakfast into him." "How so?" I asked. "Why, he is a better dog; he runs better, scents better, barks better, and comes in at night in better shape. And then, if we walk home, he gets pretty well rested and has his 'breakfast' before a great while; or, if we ride, he has it as soon as we get home; and (if it is cold weather) I let him lie in the sitting-room an hour or two after he eats, and then he will go to his kennel and sleep all night, and *without trembling*; and he turns out next morning in good shape for another tramp, if called on." "Do you 'fix' yourself in the same manner?" I could but ask. "Not *much*," he replied; "I eat before I start, and take a lunch along; but I don't know but the old dog has the best of it, after all." As a matter of fact, the aged dog is like a sprightly youth still, while his master, at middle-age, is a decrepit old man.

[65] This is a characteristic of most hunting dogs—not the exception. It is not that they know more about dietetics than their masters, for I do not think they do, but, gluttons as they are, they "rather hunt than eat."

The importance of rest after meals has never been fully appreciated by people in general. Even those who advocate the need of it, have usually,—perhaps because of the difficulties in the way of demanding more,—asked for only a half, or a whole hour; while it is the popular belief that "exercise after eating promotes digestion," and the fact is cited that Sunday is, to the laborer, the worst day of all the week,—a day of leisure, affording ample time for digestion, if that is all that is required. But that is not all. The "bad feeling" which comes on after the second meal on Sunday—the "Sunday headache," of which so many complain—results from the radical change of habit from the six days of hard labor: accustomed as he is to digesting a large part of his three meals together, at night, after he has *earned* them, physiologically speaking,—that is, after his labor has provided the digestive fluids in the blood, by means of which his food is dissolved, and made ready for absorption into the circulation,—when Sunday, with its leisure, and possibly even more than usually excessive indulgence, comes, instead of having the blood diverted to the general muscular system, as the result of active labor, it is called to the stomach and the circulation becomes overcharged with nutritive material. Hence lethargy, tendency to sleep, headache, etc.

The fact is,

EXERCISE AFTER EATING

by *preventing* digestion, often delays or modifies the ill-feeling which would otherwise be experienced shortly after over-indulgence at the table. Hence gentle exercise in the open air will prove the least of two evils; an emetic, the best of all remedies. The liquids[66] being to a great extent absorbed, plethora is prevented or delayed because the solids remain undigested in the stomach! But this solid residue, favored by the internal temperature, begins to ferment, after a time, and causes more or less irritation and congestion of the mucous lining of the stomach, which gives rise to the sensation popularly called "hunger"; and thus every few hours, and when the patient impatiently awaits the call to dinner and thinks himself most in need of food, he is, in fact, in the very worst condition to take it. Ninety-five persons in every hundred have this disease (for it is nothing less than chronic dyspepsia) throughout life. The fact that the meal affords immediate relief argues nothing against this position; it is the seventy-five or eighty per cent. of water contained in and taken with the meal that relieves the congestion. It forms a poultice, so to say, for the congested mucous membrane of the stomach; but unfortunately it can not, as when applied externally upon a throbbing sore thumb, for example, be removed when it becomes dry. We see this disease at its worst in infancy, when meals are most frequent and excessive.

[66] In case of an ordinary "mixed meal," water composes something near four-fifths of all; solids, pure and simple, one-fifth. Even roast beef is about three-fourths water, and vegetables the same.

Jules Virey settled the question, as it seems to me, regarding the effects of work after eating. He took two dogs of same size, age, and general *physique*; gave both a fast-day, and then treated them to a square meal, alike in quantity and variety. One was sent to his kennel, while the other was permitted to follow the carriage which conveyed the doctor on his rounds. After the coach-dog had had two hours and a half of (not vigorous, but gentle) exercise, and immediately on his return, the doctor had both dogs slain and dissected. The kennel-dog had thoroughly digested his breakfast,—not a trace of it was found in his stomach,—while with the other, the work of digestion had not even begun; the mutton cubes and potato chips remained intact, precisely as when first eaten. It is evident from this that the rule, "Never eat until you have leisure to digest,"[67] is a good one, and that for a hard-working person (what man or woman works as hard as the enthusiastic hunting-dog?) the one-meal-a-day system would often prove the best,—indeed, in some instances, this would be the only means of preventing sickness. We may not know in how many instances the laborer digests his breakfast, dinner, and supper together (or about all that he does digest) after he is in bed for the night. Any approach to such a state is provocative of disease.

[67] It by no means follows that the man of all leisure, or the "loafer," can, because of abundant rest after meals, digest the large quantity of food he may be tempted to swallow. On the contrary, he probably does not digest one-fourth of it. The balance is assuredly retained to work him injury at last. No man really *digests*, speaking strictly, in excess of the physiological needs of his organism; the fact that one man "carries off," so to speak, an immense amount of food without apparent or immediate inconvenience, argues simply that he has greater excretory capacity—perhaps was endowed originally with a greater degree of vitality—than another who is constantly troubled though eating less and working more. Persons of the latter class still exceed their normal amount; hence their digestive troubles.

The dyspeptic's dreams, which disturb his sleep, rob him of needed rest, and often cause him to wake more tired than when he went to bed, would be banished, or at least favorably modified, if, at the close of his day's work, after sufficient rest from the fatigues and cares of the day, he were to take his well-earned ration, and, after a period of recreation, if there still remained time for this, go to his bed.

Another instance I will mention, that of the man who may almost be called the father of hygiene in this country. He says: "I have tested the sufficiency of eating once in twenty-four hours [he has himself lived on this system for eleven years, and continues so to live; and has, besides, tested its advantages upon patients in certain forms of disease] and have done work enough to put a much younger man to his trumps if he had to do it. My food is very simple; I do not eat more at one meal than almost any person eats who takes three meals a day; I keep my body well built up in flesh and in vigor of muscle, considering that incurable organic difficulties render great muscular activity impracticable. I keep up my own strength, and have held in check my constitutional conditions so that I have reached old age" [72 years].

I could mention a score or more of similar instances; and, as stated elsewhere, no person ever tried the plan and found occasion for abandoning it, except from considerations utterly remote from health. In fact, under certain circumstances, as in travelling, this system is a most beneficent one; it makes a person independent of railway restaurants and lunch-counters; for at some time during the day, usually, as at night in a good hotel, one can obtain, if not always a really hygienic meal, still a comparatively good one.

With reference to the amount of food to be taken at the single meal, I have observed this: those who would be termed hearty eaters, on the three-meal system, will usually eat no more at their one meal than formerly at dinner alone; some, indeed, find much less than this suffices to sustain them in the best manner. This is largely due, however, to the superior quality of their diet, since people of this class invariably become, practically, vegetarians and, withal, use a large proportion of bread, a pure nutrient, instead of flesh, a nutro-stimulant. The amount of food taken, under any circumstances, will depend largely upon one's views as to the true office of eating.

In the case of a certain class of dyspeptics who, while going to the table three times every day, yet do not eat, all told, a single satisfactory meal; who in the entire year, perhaps, scarcely know the comfort of eating a full meal, and who live on in this manner year after year, the one-meal system would banish their nausea and lack of appetite within a reasonable time, and, in some instances, such persons would eat, and with a relish long unknown to them, more food every day than they now force down at their three or more attempts at eating. There would also result a corresponding improvement in their general health, more especially if this reform were accompanied by others, when needed, as to fresh air and exercise.

Says Dr. Nichols, of London, who speaks with knowledge, from having tested it: "The one-meal-a-day system will largely increase any person's working capacity."

Note.—One item well worth considering, especially by the laboring classes who find it so difficult to support a little family on $8 or $10 per week, while imitating the dietetic habits of their employers: Dr. T. L. Nichols, named above, experimenting as to cost of living, has lived week in and week out, in London, at a cost (for food) of sixty or eighty cents per week (taken two meals then), maintaining full vigor, and weight, and performing arduous literary labors, combined with a somewhat active mode of life. Personally, the author was never more vigorous or better fitted for hard work,—in short, better nourished,—than when living for several months on the 1-meal plan and on a diet of unleavened Graham gems and fruit, the total cost of which was less than ten cents per day.

CHAPTER XV.

THE NATURAL DIET.[68]

As the result of personal experience, my mind having been called to the subject by the successful experiment—if, indeed, it can be regarded as an experiment,—of a very intelligent and worthy family in Southern California, I am convinced that the "natural diet,"—uncooked cereals[69] and fruit,—is the diet *par excellence*, as regards strict purity, digestibility, and efficiency. Not only is much less of it required to maintain the normal weight and strength, but it is in other regards superior. One thought I will suggest, in this connection, and one which is more significant, I believe, than many persons would at first consider: raw grain, as all are aware, will "keep" indefinitely under fair conditions; while cooked, it "spoils" in a day or two. The former is more readily and more thoroughly preserved from undesirable changes in the alimentary canal; hence less liability of indigestion. Such portions of whole grain as may be swallowed without mastication, will pass on and out without danger of the putrefactive changes which result from an excess, or deficient mastication of cooked food. Regarding the gustatory pleasure to be derived from a diet of this sort, while it is less seductive to the abnormal appetite, still, even here, no individual really needing food would find this disagreeable, though reference were made solely to whole wheat, masticated with the aid of good teeth; or to the meal, mixed with nice fruit juices or the fruits themselves, when, from unnatural living, the teeth are badly decayed. Our teeth would not fail us if, from childhood, we *used* them, and our food furnished the material to build and maintain them.

[68] This subject having been treated in a most masterly manner by Prof. Schlickeysen, of Germany—considering fully the chemical and anatomical theories, and presenting the anthropological, the physiological, and the dietetical arguments so clearly and convincingly—I design here merely to give a few practical tests illustrating the advantages of a truly natural and pure diet, while recommending every devout student of this subject, every conscientious and thoughtful person to procure the work, entitled Fruit and Bread,—translated from the German by Dr. Holbrook, and published by M. L. Holbrook & Co., New York,—and read it for himself.

[69] Even as late as the time of the Roman republic, the baking or other cooking of grain was regarded as injurious. When the grains are first broken, but not finely ground, they may be eaten with fruit, if one gradually accustom himself to it. Let it not be said that this is going too far, for in the recognition and application of truth we can not go too far; rather have those gone too far who have deviated from this method. The difference between pure cracked wheat and the bread is always considerable. The bread consumes in its digestion [a part of] the power which itself supplies, while the wheat not only nourishes, but, like fresh fruit, *increases the vital strength.—Fruit and Bread*, p. 163.

"The vitality stored up in uncooked plants and fruits is greatly impaired by all our culinary processes."—*Ibid.*, p. 116.

"Animals in a state of nature, subsisting upon their own chosen foods, are capable of fully digesting the nutritive elements, leaving only an inoffensive residue, while the unsuitable character of human foods is sufficiently indicated by the horrible and disease-breeding product which they yield. —*Ibid.*"

"Uncooked fruits, especially, excite the mind to its highest activity. After eating them we experience an inclination to vigorous exercise, and also an increased capacity for study and all mental work; while cooked food causes a feeling of satiety and sluggishness."—*Ibid.*

Were I to enumerate the foods at present eaten raw by all of our millions of people, less surprise would be felt by my readers at the suggestion of restricting one's diet to such articles as are agreeable in their natural state. Take, for example, apples, pears, peaches, grapes, oranges, etc.; all of the plums; bananas, dates, figs, raisins; cabbage, lettuce, celery, radishes, etc.; and to this list might well be added sweet corn, and the common variety of green corn, and peas; few people but find the latter delicious to their taste, and the corn is as much more crisp and juicy and wholesome raw than cooked, as are peaches or pears. I know individuals who were never fond of corn, would never eat it until happening to try a fresh young ear *au naturel*, who now use it freely every summer. This would be the case with very many, if not most people, if their prejudices were cast aside. I have named only a few articles of a few classes, but any one can extend the list at pleasure, adding walnuts, almonds, filberts, etc.,

etc. Unfortunately these raw foods have been commonly used as *surfeit dishes,* delicious articles that we can eat after having already over-eaten, and when more steak, potatoes, and gravy, or pastry, would, perhaps, send a shudder throughout the frame, and, often enough, when an emetic would be a more wholesome dessert than even walnuts and raisins. Let any one, first arranging for a clean stomach by skipping supper the previous night, try a breakfast consisting of a couple of bananas, one or two dozen walnuts (or any sort preferred), with a handful of nice raisins,—both the nuts and raisins being thoroughly masticated, the latter to the point of well crushing the stones,—ending, or beginning, the *seance* with oranges, and, at night, the second and last meal, of favorite fruits, beginning with a small portion of "oat groats" or wheat, (of course any other choice may be made, a dozen, or a score, indeed, from week to week,) taking care to exercise enough to "earn" his food,[70] and see if this principle of alimentation will not cure his disorders, whatever they may be. It would end the wretched business of "colds" and "hay-fever" which, according to the *Boston Herald*, a noted American divine says, "will make a man forget his God, the Bible, and everything else—but his disease." Even the common hygienic diet, so called, and abstemious living, would make such blasphemy impossible, and would make a better man of the great London preacher, for example,—Mr. Spurgeon,—who recently wrote to a friend, and, apparently without the least shamefacedness: "My old disorder has come upon me like an armed man and laid me low. I can not walk or even stand, and the pain renders it difficult to think consecutively upon any subject." And this with reference to a disorder (the gout) caused by eating and drinking unwholesomely—the injury being augmented, directly and indirectly, by the use of tobacco or wine. Mr. Spurgeon's weight is fifty, if not seventy-five pounds greater than is normal for him, considering fully his natural *physique*, and the use he makes of his muscular system. He may be in the habit of restricting his appetite; he may eat much less than most of his associates, and even be esteemed a small eater and very abstemious; nevertheless his form is gross, and he has the gout—two unimpeachable witnesses to the truth of my position.

[70] "Live on sixpence a day and earn it," was the "favorite prescription" of a famous London physician.

"We can not doubt," says Dr. Oswald, "that the highest degree of health could only be attained by strict conformity to Haller's[71] rule, *i.e.*, by subsisting exclusively on the pure and unchanged products of Nature. This view is indorsed (indirectly) in the writings of Drs. Alcott, Bernard, Schlemmer, Hall, and Dio Lewis, and directly by Schrodt, Jules Virey, and others. In the tropics such a mode of life would not imply anything like asceticism: a meal of milk and three or four kinds of sweet fruits, fresh dates, bananas, and grapes, would not clash with the still higher rule, that eating, like every other natural function, should be a pleasure and not a penance. Heat destroys the delicate flavor of many fruits, and makes others indigestible by coagulating their albumen. But," continues this authority,—and I am not disposed to dispute the soundness of the position, speaking generally (as, indeed, Dr. Oswald, himself, was speaking),—"in the frigid latitudes, where we have to dry and garner many vegetable products in order to survive the unproductive season, the process of cooking [some classes of] our food has advantages which fully outweigh such objections." To the very rational assumption that, "few men with post-diluvian teeth would agree with Dr. Schlemmer that hard grain is preferable to bread," I would reply, that for people who could not or would not grind their own grist, as do our most robust animals—well nourished, but hard-working draught or road horses—the whole-wheat meal, freshly and coarsely ground, with a light dressing of rich milk,[72] or, more wholesome still, eaten with nuts and thoroughly masticated, is more delicious than bread, even if made from the same quality of Graham. If the Graham be taken dry, with a few raisins at each mouthful, it would require a fine taste to distinguish between this and the walnuts and raisins so generally acceptable to epicures. If the milk dressing is used, it should simply be poured over the (unsifted) Graham, and not made into a batter. With a dish of Graham as described, and such fruit as can usually be obtained all the year round, either fresh or (in winter) dried, as apples, raisins, dates, figs,[73] prunes (the last, like dried apples, peaches, etc., soaked not overmuch, but until tender), one may make a meal sufficiently delicious, and at the same time absolutely pure—if the *milk* is derived from a healthy creature. And here I would remark, that although cow's milk is a strictly natural food for the calf only, still, if the cow be properly fed (not "driven,"[74] as is the custom in dairies) and the milk properly cared for—kept free from air vitiated by the emanations of decaying vegetables, meats, or other source of impurity, but *open*[75] in a pure atmosphere—few need abstain altogether from this most delicious food. Nevertheless, no one may feel at liberty to *drink* milk copiously, as water: calves, babies, etc., whose natural food it is, take it slowly and "chew" it thoroughly! We may well take a hint from this. (See Biliousness.)

[71] Albrecht Von Haller, M.D., F.R.S., the father of the science of physiology, born at Berne, Oct. 18, 1708; ... practiced medicine with great applause at Berne, 1729-36; ... became physician to the King of England 1739. He was a voluminous writer on physiology, anatomy, botany, surgery, and practical medicine; author of ... almost an incredible number of reviews and scientific papers. His hypotheses were ... admirable for their scientific spirit, and for the great stimulus which they gave to physiological study throughout Europe.—*Encyclopedia.*

[72] See note 4 in Appendix, p. 280.

[73] These three—raisins, dates, figs,—containing as they do in their natural state, about 14, 58 and 62 per cent., respectively, of sugar, require no addition of saccharine matters to "preserve" them; and, accordingly, they constitute, as we find them in the market, a perfectly natural and wholesome food, taken in due proportion, with grain and the various nuts.

[74] A phrase used to describe the process of feeding excessively to produce an abnormal flow of milk. Under this practice the cows soon become tuberculous ("consumptive"); and it is said that they become useless after three or four years, on an average: they are "driven to death," unless disposed of just prior to their decline. Nursing mothers often suffer from this disease, while the infant fattens and becomes sick from overfeeding.

[75] Kept in a close vessel, milk soon becomes foul; and after being thus enclosed requires considerable stirring to aerate it, when it again acquires its normal flavor. Cistern water treated to an occasional deep stirring will remain sweet; and when the water in a cistern has become devitalized for want of air simply, it can be reclaimed readily in the above manner.

In making the change from cooked to uncooked food, the unassisted novice will experience more or less inconvenience, usually; and this will arise from one of three causes; perhaps two or even all three causes will combine to create the uneasiness (and indigestion, even, sometimes) experienced: (1) the stomach, adapted, so far as possible, to the digestion of cooked foods, requires some time (and experience or practice) to adapt itself to the new order of things,[76] hence indigestion, varied in extent according (*a*) to the abruptness of the change, and (*b*) the quantity of the new food taken; (2) accustomed to distention from the bulky character of the old diet, if only a physiological ration of the pure and more nutritious food be swallowed, the stomach misses the stimulus of distention: time will be required (in some cases) for the stomach to remodel itself as regards *size* —unless a large proportion of fruit[77] is used in conjunction with the cereals. Some dyspeptics, to be sure, by their "mincing" diet occasioned by nausea and lack of appetite, seem to have reduced the size of their stomachs, even below the normal dimensions of that organ; (3) the uncooked grain being more nutritious than the bread formed from it (and especially than bread made from wheat *starch*—"white bread"), one may readily take an overdose if the wheat *meal* be used and dressed with milk; but if the whole grain be employed he will be content with a modest ration; the new exercise of chewing—putting the teeth to their normal use—soon wearies the muscles of the face, and he will be tempted to pass to the "second course"—the fruit—quite early in the engagement. The amount of grain food necessary to thoroughly nutrify the body, is comparatively small. In the form of bread, we are apt to eat altogether too much. But given pure food, and each individual may be safely left to decide the proportion of grain, fruit, and water to suit his own case; the point is to maintain strength and avoid flatulence, and all other symptoms of indigestion.

[76] It has been observed that cows are temporarily affected adversely by *any* change from their established diet—give less milk, *at first*, when grain is *added* to their pasture rations, as well as when they are deprived of an accustomed feed of grain. "The effect is due to the action of the stomach, to adapt its character to the digestion of an established food. The food may change suddenly, but the action of the stomach can only change slowly, and hence defective digestion follows."—(*National Live Stock Journal*). With humans, as has been already remarked, a change from a very unwholesome to the purest system of diet may, at first, result in defective digestion; but if the change be made discreetly the final result will assuredly be as satisfactory as that which follows a favorable modification of the cow's diet.

[77] Whenever, in making the change under consideration, flatulency or pressure at the kidney follows the use of fruit, the quantity habitually taken should be lessened. There is a temptation always to continue the habitual distention of the stomach by the use of too much fruit at first. The system accustomed to a small amount of fruit, can not immediately adapt itself to an unusual quantity: *all* changes should be somewhat gradual, not necessarily by the continued use of any unwholesome substance, but with relation to the *manner of adopting the new regimen.*

At the world-famed "Grape Cures" (for dyspepsia and its sequel, consumption), the diet during "the season," consists almost exclusively of ripe grapes: the patients stroll about the vineyards, and pick and eat. During the balance of the year the diet is composed chiefly of fruit, with a portion of cooked cereals. But we may obtain a more definite lesson from the experience of Mr. and Mrs. Hinde and their children.

For nearly five years, this family, consisting of father, mother, and four children, have lived on this truly natural diet. They are very intellectual and refined people. Their home is in Southern California. They have enjoyed typical health during these five years; the mother, indeed, recovered her health by means of this diet, having failed, under medical treatment, to obtain relief from serious disorders which would be popularly and medically described as "incident to her sex," but which, when they exist, are everywhere and always incident to *violation of law*. Every trace of her disorder disappeared during this lady's first year of living on uncooked food and outdoor air, and no vestige of her "weaknesses" has returned. The members of this family all live very active lives; they take two meals,—morning and afternoon,—a small amount of the cereals, and a large proportion of fruit of various kinds. Our national pastime-luncheon, the ubiquitous peanut, forms a part of their regular dietary. It is a very nutritious vegetable, and, certainly, if agreeable enough, as we know it is, to take a prominent part in the sensual enjoyment of a very large class, who feel that life is not worth living unless much of their leisure time is spent in palate-tickling, it can not be sneered at as "one of the 'messes' of those peculiar people," (formerly a common remark about hygienists, some of whom have, without doubt, advocated an unnatural asceticism.) I will make a few brief extracts from letters written by the lady in question, at, and after the time I was living on uncooked food. As will be seen, the work was altogether new to me, and I went astray at first, regarding the proportions of grain and fruit: "Your cupful of grain," she writes, "is more than double what my husband takes, and I use still less; but we eat very much more fresh fruit than you do." ... "I had intended to say in my last letter, that some people object to so much cold food, especially in the morning. I did not at all like it myself, at first, being always used to 'a good cup of tea' the first thing; however, use soon becomes second nature, and I prefer it now. In winter, when the apples or melons seem really cold, I bring them to a moderately cold temperature by warming slightly—the same with tomatoes: of these last, quite a lot have ripened up, although it is mid-winter, (Feb. 6, '81.) We find that *too much nut*-food causes indigestion,[78] and it is better to combine a little vegetable-food always, if possible." ... "One little incident in our lives here, may interest you: our oldest daughter, aged 13, has just been on a visit to some friends—the family of a doctor of the old school. His wife remarked one day that she liked the uncooked food very much, and would always use it, only she ate 'what the others did, to keep them company.' Alice replied (and you may imagine how proud I felt when it was repeated to me by the doctor's daughter), 'I am sure you do not understand the importance of it, then!' You would be surprised to see how firm the children are: they could not, by any kind of bribery, I believe, be induced to swerve one iota from the true principles upon which we live, and they have been severely tested, too." I regret to say that a year after the above was written, these people decided to test once more the influence of cooking their food; although it may furnish valuable evidence, and I predict their return to the natural diet with renewed faith. Now (Sept. 1, 1882), after a few months' use of artificially prepared food (their diet is still very simple; they use no animal food, nor fancy dishes, no pastry, nor *hot* drinks), such sentences as the following are quite significant: "Well, both my husband and myself think it possible there may be more 'ailments' from the use of cooked food, but there is more enjoyment too, and we shall have to take the bitter and the sweet together." ... "I know it [uncooked food] increases the spiritual perceptions greatly."[79]... "I still believe it would be a sure preventive of disease; but few, however, are prepared to adopt such an extreme mode of living." Once more: "The experiment has done us good, I am sure; and I feel glad of the lessons I have learned through it. I don't think I shall ever be what I was before using it." [*i. e.*, sickly]. Of this we can, of course, judge better later on. From an earlier letter, written in January (the 30th), 1881, and while they were enjoying the natural diet for the fourth year, I make a few extracts: "Its effects are truly wonderful, and far exceed my expectations.... The sequel has proved that it not only ensures health to those already healthy, but eradicates former weaknesses when these exist; for instance, rheumatism and 'sciatica,' from which I used to suffer—both have left me, I think never to return. The children frequently suffered with toothache, and occasionally with earache; now they are never troubled. I believe the hot food destroys the teeth, and renders the body generally more susceptible of taking colds. I used to take cold on the slightest exposure; now I don't know what it is to have one. And sore throat was sure to follow a cold; now I am quite exempt, and have been for two years."[80]

[78] The oily nuts are nutritious, and a small proportion, only, should be eaten; except in cold weather.

[79] I desire to call the attention and fasten it for a moment upon this feature of the case.

[80] With reference to the prophylactic and curative effects of this diet I quote from "Vegetarian Life in Germany: *A Paper, by a Lady Member of the German Vegetarian Society, read 15th Jan., 1881, at Manchester England, and reprinted by request.*"

"Others, especially those whose occupations afford little or no exercise, as writers, artists, official persons, etc., prefer from time to time to live upon fruits alone, in order to clear their blood and thus prevent illness. Dr. Richard Nagel, of Burman, was one of the first to try such a cure, and with brilliant success. As he is a learned man, and his health rules are accepted by most German vegetarians, I take the liberty to give you an abridged translation of them:

"I. Take often during the day a drink of pure cool fresh water; rain-water is best. Vegetarians who live plainly and upon fruits only, have very little thirst.

"II. Wash the whole body with cool fresh water every morning before breakfast; poor-blooded persons may use in winter a little warm, but never hot water.

"III. All kinds of sweet fruits and roots are to be commended in an uncooked form. These are so nourishing that we can live upon fruit alone. (Dr. Nagel, himself, so lived in 1871, from February 25th to April 7th, that is during forty-one winter days, and you know that our German winter is much colder than yours. During this time he was extremely well, and worked hard as a physician and writer)."

Further on, and after describing the two-years-old baby's remarkable health and perfect appetite: "He never causes me the least trouble; is always ready to eat a good breakfast, taking just what we do, and is truly a marvel of sweet infant life." After a brief reference to the persecutions received from their neighbors at the first: ... "But that is nothing; we have lived it all down, and we are in better health to-day, all of us, than any family about, for many a mile. Why, they are all complaining of *colds* now, and yet we have the loveliest climate and the most delightful atmosphere under the sun. We never have any colds, or neuralgia, or rheumatism. Whatever may be said in derision of our diet, and, of course, there are more or less remarks, we have the best of it anyway; and, oh, the load of expense, labor and care and anxiety that is removed! The children are harmonious and happy, devoting their spare time to useful pursuits—we all have so much more spare time now," etc., etc.

From another letter:

"... But I must hasten to answer your queries. 1st. As to how we prepare our food in winter. We have apples, raisins, oranges, and figs, which need no preparation. Wheat and rye we grind first in a large mill and finish off in a spice mill, and usually eat it dry with juicy fruits. I can eat rye, apples, nuts, and raisins, and make a good meal. We confine ourselves to what we raise here, chiefly because we think it best. We raise our own peanuts, and if you will take them *unroasted*, and grind with your grain, you will get a very palatable, strengthening food, alone or with raisins; they contain a very sweet oil which, as we learn, is beginning to be appreciated in England. I prefer the peanuts in this form because they need to be very finely masticated. I can work longer after such a breakfast and not feel hungry than anything else I have tried. We have delicious musk-melons now, also water-melons, but the latter are deteriorating, being out of season. Our ripe tomatoes are nearly over; after these are gone we shall use our dried peaches, pears, and apples, merely soaked in cold water until soft—not sloppy. We use rain-water in winter. I make a salad for dinner, often, as follows: lettuce washed and cut small, a few ripe tomatoes peeled and cut up, and one or two green peppers cut fine; pouring over a dressing of raisin syrup, made by soaking black raisins for twenty-four hours, and straining. This salad I vary by substituting celery for lettuce. I assure you it is a most healthful dish, and so sweet and nice with rye. We use oatmeal soaked for twelve hours in just enough water to soften it, and then well beaten; with either raisins [grapes] or dried fruits it is very delicious. I did not at first like rye, but after a little we all came to regard it the sweetest grain we have. The children are very fond of cauliflower—just the flour part—and green pease, fresh-picked are a great dish with us. Some like radishes and garden cress and a few things of that nature. I prefer fruits with my grain, and we can have them fresh, of some sort, all the year round. Strawberries come in about March—indeed, we have a few even now [February]. I'm going to make a 'natural fruitcake,' this week, for our little girl's birthday. I shall send a piece by post to Mrs. Page, with full directions for making it. We had one at New Year's, and even those who live on cooked food pronounced it 'as good as they ever tasted.' But very little of our time, however, is taken up, usually, with the preparation of our food; only, on special occasions, we amuse ourselves a little in such ways, for the children's sake. At all times, however, we have a good variety of food; in fact, too much, I sometimes think. We eat more in quantity than others, but a large proportion is fruit, which furnishes all our liquid food except fresh water. We all enjoy our food *thoroughly*; the children never ask for anything between meals [two meals only], only baby comes as regularly as possible for an apple at half-past eleven—of course he gets it."

The following letter from a veteran hygienist refers to the family whose history I have been relating.

My dear Dr. Page:

Your letter of February 13th, enclosing letters from Mr. and Mrs. Hinde for us to read and to make extracts from for *The Laws*, came duly to hand. I have read them with great interest, for they do but add to my conviction that, as yet, the divinely ordained mode of living for man on earth has received, in the minds of so-called hygienists, small conception, and in the life of the best of us comparatively poor illustration, and, therefore, just such experience as these dear people are having in their search for better methods of realizing, developing, and making serviceable spiritual power are of great interest to me. They always have been.

It has been a matter of great regret with me, that being an incurably diseased man, and being shut up to the necessity of working up, to the best degree possible for me, a revolution in the thought and conduct of people at large, in matters pertaining to their life on earth, I have not been able physically nor circumstantially to carry out my life as I have wanted to do. I have done some things, but always under circumstances that endangered my available power to live and work, while making such transitions as I was determined to make.

I have settled several principles which enter as constituent elements into the philosophy of life of the human organism. Among them I may mention two: One is, the changes from bad to good, or from worse to better, can never be made reconstructively, except under the policy which governs construction. Now, as all growth of any living organism, or any part of it, is, relatively speaking, slow, so all reparation of any injured part in such organism relatively has to be slow. Reconstruction, therefore, is slow if according to law. This of itself speaks condemningly of the system of drug medication, because everywhere do drug doctors seek to produce changes from bad to good, or from worse to better, rapidly. This is unphilosophical, and, therefore, can be, on the whole, only open to criticism as being bad practice.

Another is, that where morbid conditions have existed until they have become chronic, and the organism has become adjusted thereto, changes from the abnormal to the normal can not be made without aggravation of those conditions. I have never known a person to go from chronic derangements of any organ in his body to normal conditions of it, without passing through an acute stage,[81] and this acute stage is critical in its nature, subjecting the organ to added liability for the time, may be subjecting the whole organism to it. Thousands of persons die every day under medical treatment in this country from badly-managed critical changes through which they have to pass.

[81] This was illustrated in the case of Mrs. Hinde, who says of her first experience: "I fully expected suffering as a consequence, and so there was for a time; but it proved a blessing in disguise."—AUTHOR.

Thirdly, I am satisfied that of all the diseases with which doctors have to deal, and of which persons die, ninety-five per cent. of them have their origin in bad dietetic indulgence, and in deviations from right way of living, caused directly by, and to be attributed to, bad habits of eating and drinking. If you take a hundred diseases, as they are called, and study the predisposing and the provoking causes to their production, you will find that at least ninety-five per cent. have their origin in derangements of the stomach and the organs that are in direct sympathy with it.

I take it upon me to say on my platform very frequently, and I repeat the same as I would repeat it from any public platform if I were talking to a public audience: Give me the right and the power, by and with the consent of any given population, whether one thousand or one million, to control their dietetic conditions, and I will take care of their diseases, and, in less than the life of a generation, will banish from their midst seven-eighths of all the diseases now common to physicians in their practice; will stop the diseases, and deaths that grow out of a prevalence of these diseases and their methods of treatment; will put an end to the vices and the crimes everywhere extant, and which it is so difficult for society and government to manage, and thoroughly revolutionize the physical and moral status of such people.

We have to go to the bottom of things in order to get to the top of things, for the home of the eternal righteousness is so high that no ladder can reach it, unless its lower end rests on bed-rock. Who builds his house on quicksand runs the risk of his life. Who climbs to the skies by any false means of ascent that he may seek to establish, will find his fate foreshadowed in the simple fact that he does not commence his ascent from a secure foundation.

Yours very truly,
JAMES C. JACKSON.

Mr. Isaac B. Rumford, and son, hard-working farmers, of Bakersfield, Cal., have lived strictly on the "natural diet" for upwards of two years. Mr. Rumford has been a chronically-diseased man for many years; now, however, he is so far improved as to be able to do, as he says, "a good day's work." "It is doing for me," he writes, "what I have been seeking and sorrowing after, vainly until now, for twenty years—giving me health. My son also finds it a perfect diet, and would not readily exchange it for any other; indeed, we both enjoy our food more than formerly on the old system. By another year," he adds, "I shall be able to give you still more information on this subject, as others are beginning to be impressed with the advantages of this regimen." (See Appendix.)

A. R. B., of New York city, has lived chiefly on uncooked grain and fruit for upwards of a year; and his young wife, also, has tried it to a considerable extent. Two years ago Mrs. B. was threatened with consumption, and was told by her physician that unless she changed her diet (she was then beginning the vegetarian regimen) she would certainly not live a year. She "needed meat and milk in abundance," he said. But she only lived the more abstemiously, and on coarse bread, with fruit, chiefly, and, during the past year, has eaten considerable uncooked "bread," and all symptoms of her disease have disappeared. Mr. B. had nasal catarrh; but this has disappeared, and he now finds himself thoroughly nourished and better able than ever before to perform his duties. His diet consists of two meals,—7 A.M. and 6 P.M.,—and with but little variation, the two combined make about a half cupful each, wheat and oat groats, with five or six nice apples. His appetite has become sufficiently normal to enable him to enjoy this diet fully. This is in winter. In summer less grain and more fruit.

As bearing upon the supposed difficulties in the way of introducing the natural diet, should any choose to adopt it, I can not forbear relating a little incident of recent occurrence: For some weeks past, I have been living exclusively, and with great satisfaction, upon this diet. In a conversation upon the subject, a friend expressed, along with some surprise at my statements as to the gustatory pleasures of this diet and its completeness for nutrifying the body, a curiosity to know just how it would seem to sit down to a meal without a single dish of cooked food, nor any odor of smoking viands about. "Very good," I said, "dine with us to-morrow, and bring the children." This he promised, and on the following day, Sunday, he came up with his two children, a boy of seven and a girl of three years. Nothing was said to them by their father before, nor by any one after their arrival, as to the kind of food to be set before them, they were simply invited out to dinner, and anticipated a good time. The injudicious comments, or "chaffing," of parents and friends, will very easily "set" children against what would naturally be their own inclinations if given a fair chance, without having their minds prejudiced, I mean, by the notions, or the dyspeptic idiosyncracies of their elders. At 4 P.M. the table was set, but with no extras on account of company, although here "extras" would imply no additional trouble nor, perhaps, expense. There were dates,—"Persian," or the kind which are in regular tiers and handled comfortably,—walnuts, filberts, raisins, a variety of apples, and, for bread, a fruit-dish containing "oat groats." The latter was served as the first course, the children eating of this natural bread with every appearance of satisfaction, as did all the company, a few teaspoonfuls each. All united in calling it sweet and good. Then came walnuts and raisins; some added filberts, others took only the latter, after which, dates, and then, for dessert, apples; of these, one or two each were eaten. In the midst of the nuts and raisins, I may add, and what surprised my visitor more than all else, both children *asked*, voluntarily, for "a few more oats," which they received and ate with a gusto! As we arose from the table, my friend (a banker, by the way, and a "good liver,") said, "There, I can truly say that I have never eaten a more satisfactory dinner; taken all in all, this has been a model meal." "How about the children?" I asked, of him, but they answered; "I have had a splendid dinner," said the boy. "I've had a splendid dinner," chorused the little three-year-old. The father added (what was in my own mind), that he enjoyed the meal all the more because of the non-necessity for restricting the children in any manner: there was no occasion for caution—no "mustn't eat so fast," no "I'm afraid you are not chewing your food thoroughly," "No, dear, no more of the preserves,—they will hurt you," nor any nuisance of the sort; nor any risk in consequence; and I remarked, with my friend's entire acquiescence, that, often as I had observed them, both in their home and at my own table, never had I seen them so apparently satisfied in every respect, from the beginning to the end of a meal; that, in fact, they had never enjoyed a meal in so utterly unrestricted a manner; and at the same time, they arose from the table with no indication of surfeit—no heaviness, nor succeeding sleepiness or peevishness, as we often witness with children after an ordinary dinner.

Here was a delicious and ample midwinter dinner for six at a total cost of less than the meat alone for a mixed meal,—with no brewing, baking or fuming-up the home, or heating up and using up its mistress in the preparation, and clearing away of the meal, not to mention the other injurious effects of an ordinary "company dinner." A few weeks later, in response to an invitation from my little guests, I had the pleasure of a return-dinner of the same sort, and a Christmas (1882) dinner at that, at which a larger company assembled, and all pronounced it complete; and the servants did not complain of being overworked—nor underfed. One of these was overheard to say, "*Dessert*'s good enough for me!"

I would ask all prudent parents, Are you not often disturbed about the little ones' diet—about the pie, cake, pudding, etc., and are they not frequently made ill by "over-indulgence," as it is called, in these things? How can you expect a little, growing child, with an appetite like that of a shark (if hot, melting viands, or artificial sweets are before them), with no sort of physiological knowledge, in fact a normal and proper disgust for anything of the sort, no idea of prudence, but only a dread of your frequent and necessary cautions,—how can you expect a child, with mouth full of hot bread,—or any bread,—with butter, milk, or sauce, or mashed potatoes, garnished with gravy turkey, stuffing, and cranberry, all melting in his mouth, to "chew" what requires no chewing and can not be made wholesome by chewing, and "hold" what will rush away into the stomach as though impelled by an all-controlling force? It can not be done, you can not do it yourselves, and as for the young ones, it is the refinement of cruelty to attempt it;—it means dissatisfaction, discomfort, and, often, the destruction of what should be a happy season, to be perpetually badgering them about it; it is unnatural and wrong. Give your children the sort of food you think best for them, and let them enjoy it. If this can not be done with safety, the fault is with the food, not with them.

The best way to effect a change in an obnoxious law, as has been well said, is to enforce the law. The same principle holds in diet: If you find that you are furnishing a sort of food which, eaten unrestrictedly and in their own way, makes your children sick or endangers their health, give them something better. At the meal of which I have been speaking, there was no restraint, no cautions, nor occasion for any: the food was of that strictly natural sort which, while requiring to be well masticated, itself enforced the law. The sharp teeth of the children cut the oats perfectly; there was no stimulation, nor temptation to hurry the food into the stomach without masticating it, no feverish appetency, as with hot, highly-seasoned viands—all wanted to chew the food as much as it "wanted to be" chewed, and, consequently, no appreciable amount of it entered the stomach unprepared for stomach-digestion. For the first time in the lives of these children, since they were weaned, could this be said of them. It can not be said of a single child in America, or elsewhere, who sits at a table supplied with ordinary food. What results from this unnatural manner of alimentation? Indigestion, inevitably, indicated by various symptoms, as, for example, flatulency which is popularly regarded as entirely natural, the odorous emanations from the younger fry being considered evidence of indiscretion instead of what it really is—disease. And what from this? Blood-poisoning, as surely; with aches, pains, feverish spells, with influenza (popularly called "a cold"), which, as can not be too much emphasized, is, strictly speaking, instead of a disease, the effort of Nature to "cure" a disease which otherwise would become so deep-seated as to demand a "run of fever" to eliminate it, and all manner of physical ailments.

I am often asked, What constitutes the scrofulous diathesis, so called, or the scrofulous "taint" supposed to be the inheritance of so many of the children of our times? My reply is this: Scrofulous persons are those, mainly, perhaps it should be said wholly, who from current bad habits (as to diet, air, and all the requirements, or any part of them, which are necessary for the maintenance of health), manufacture bad, instead of pure blood. Such persons become more and more depraved, and incapacitated for bequeathing to their offspring great vital power. In consequence the children of such parents are endowed with a feeble organism; that is, an organism incapable, at least until virtually, or nearly as possible made over new, of putting forth in any direction a great degree of force, whether of the voluntary muscular system, the brain, the digestive or excretory systems, or what not. Children of this stamp may, they often do, exhibit precocity in one or another direction—being unbalanced, so to say—and may evince much alertness, both in muscle and brain, but they soon tire: it will always be found that they are incapable of prolonged effort in any direction, without exhaustion. They may develop a fondness for study and for play, but in neither direction have they any staying power: they are *called* over-ambitious, often; they *are* undernourished always. And this, not because they do not swallow a large quantity of food (though some children are kept so surfeited as to have little relish for food, and may, consequently, eat but little, being all the time a few days ahead of their stomachs, so to say), but generally because, of all the food swallowed, not enough is digested and assimilated to sustain them, and keep them in a vigorous state. They are, like all animals, when not suffering from nausea or lack of appetite through somebody's fault, very ambitious in the way of eating; having—not inherited—but rather, I should say, *acquired* during the involuntary cramming of infancy—that special school for gluttony, which graduates near thirty per cent. of its pupils into premature graves before their first year is ended—and the injudicious feeding of the survivors in childhood, a full, perhaps rounded measure of appetency, especially for the very things which scrofulous children, of all born children, should not have. They may be greedy for study and for food (though often enough, excess of the latter makes them listless and unfit for either study or play), but have for neither, sufficient capacity for digestion and assimilation, to make them either learned or strong. It follows, if they are fed like their robust fellows who can bear up under the burden, that by reason of quality, frequency, and amount of food eaten, no portion, not even such wholesome articles as fruit, vegetables, etc., as they may have in abundance,—no portion of their food is properly digested and assimilated. It is unnatural in variety, is prepared and eaten unnaturally, and, as has been said, there ensues, as surely as any effect is simultaneous with its cause, indigestion, blood-poisoning, and the *current, daily manufacture* of "scrofulous humors," if people choose to call them by that name; and but for its misleading tendency, as at present interpreted, this name would answer as well as any. Of *pure food*, these children can digest and assimilate a given amount—an amount, indeed, suited to their peculiar needs; the balance, including *all* unwholesome substances,[82] is so much for influenza, catarrh, "scrofula," measles, "nervousness," fractiousness, ("measly disposition" was not originally a slang phrase by any means) scarlet fever, skin, scalp, and all other so-called diseases. The remedy, then, for the disorders of children of scrofulous, or any other diathesis, is plain: stop feeding them unnaturally, and feed them naturally. And the earlier in their lives this is done, and the more faithfully it is attended to, the more likely they will be to "outgrow their inheritance." I do not hesitate to say that, of those weakly-born or "tainted" children who die in infancy or childhood, or live sickly lives, in a very large proportion of cases they could, by right treatment, chiefly as to fresh air and diet, be built up above the plain of disease, *i.e.*, placed upon the highest level possible to *them*, and enabled to live fairly long lives, a comfort to themselves and a benefit to the world. And this, too, in a majority of instances, on a rigidly abstemious vegetable diet, reserving the "natural diet" for the most critical cases, or the most conscientious persons.[83]

[82] I include cream among the forbidden animal fats, especially for scrofulous subjects, for the reason that in practice I have never observed other than ultimately injurious effects from its use. I can account for this only upon the ground that if *milk* is a proper food for man, *whole* milk—like whole wheat, whole apples, whole grapes, whole beets, instead of white flour, cider, wine and sugar—only can be thus classed. The fact that many, even robust persons, can not use milk at all, and a still larger proportion cream, whereas skimmed milk is well borne by them and in some instances seems to produce lasting good effects, may be accounted for, perhaps, in the following manner: As our cows are bred and fed, their milk is abnormally loaded with fatty matters, and when skimmed, after sitting twelve or more hours, still contains, as compared with *natural* cows' milk, a full proportion of cream. Therefore, by removing the excess of cream, which is of an excretory nature, we are doing all in our power to "restore the balance," or to make the milk natural. Let those who choose make use of this delicious scum; but its administration to sick people, though often, like drugs, producing stimulating, and apparently beneficial effects, will, in the end, like every form of stimulation, hinder, if not prevent recovery. (See Stimulation.)

[83] See note 5 in Appendix, p. 281.

Finally, to add so large a line of proper foods to our dietary by a correct understanding of their real office and value—taking them out of the category of mere pastime-lunches—should, from any point of view, be accounted a great gain. We are made by that much more independent, in being elevated above the otherwise some-time-necessity of eating unmitigatedly bad, or badly-prepared food, or of going without any; for almost any corner grocery will furnish a better bill-of-fare than one often finds at poor hotels or restaurants; besides, this class of foods may be taken along better than any other: they are the most comfortable to transport and to handle *en route*, and will "keep." Moreover, they demand less time for "preliminary digestion" after eating; if, indeed, one may not, after a judicious meal of them, resume ordinary mental or muscular labor with impunity. The effect of a light lunch of fruits, is really, when one is once accustomed to their use, exhilarating to both the brain and the muscular system—stimulating, not as with a spur, but, rather, a "push behind"; or, more truly, by increase of actual strength through pabulum supplied to the blood, of a character, as I am convinced, unlike that of any form of cooked food.

Note.—In concluding this theme, while expressing the belief that this will be the diet of the future—that advancing civilization will demand it, on the score of economy, as relates to time, care, and health, no less than the comparatively trifling consideration of money cost (and yet what an item even this would be to the toiling millions!), and above all in view of the emancipation of woman from the serfdom of the kitchen, where she now exhausts herself to the injury of the family, her incessant kitchen labors tending especially to unfit her for the production of robust children—yet I would not chill the health-seeker of to-day, by insisting upon the vital importance of *every* one's breaking away abruptly from *all* present customs as regards the selection and preparation of food. To a considerable degree the usage of generations has, beyond question, adapted our systems to the use of cooked foods—has even rendered them somewhat unadapted to the *instant* use of uncooked foods—so that a radical and complete change, abruptly made, would result in temporary digestive disturbance, which (however advantageous the results of the change, finally, if persisted in with faith and courage) would render it impracticable for some persons, more especially since this temporary physical inconvenience would be added to the social inconvenience arising from placing oneself so markedly at variance with all about him. No one can form a just opinion of this last item until he attempts a radical change in his dietetic habits: it presents the greatest check imaginable to rapid progress in this direction.

A reform, however, which is at the same time feasible and, in most instances, sufficient, speaking generally,—and which, as elsewhere remarked, already has its hundreds of thousands of adherents in this country alone,—would be the adoption of the "fruit and bread," or the ordinary vegetarian diet even—banishing all doubtful dishes, condiments, spices, hot drinks—stimulants all—making a lunch (or two, even) in the course of the day, of fruit, with a biscuit or two at one of them, perhaps; and at eve, when the tired ones are rested, a regular "full meal," consisting of various bread dishes—wheat, corn, rye and oatmeal, with various admixtures of the same, which may well furnish a different flavor (several, indeed) for every day in the month—fruit, milk (for those with whom it "agrees"), vegetables and nuts. Following *this direction*, and aiming constantly, but *comfortably*, to maintain the balance between diet and labor—between the food eaten and the needs of the organism for nutriment—one may not only enjoy, as he ought, the pleasures of the table, but, in very many cases, absolutely and largely increase these pleasures, in the aggregate, considering, more especially, his exemption from sickness with its occasional involuntary fasts, and with many, the quite frequent periods of slight, or non-satisfaction, through nausea and lack of appetite arising from an injudicious dietary. This regimen lessens by one-half the housewife's burdens, as well as the cost of living, while it adds immeasurably to her health and that of her household.

CHAPTER XVI.

MALARIA—SEWER GAS.

These are very vicious companions, and cause a deal of mischief. The scientists have much to say of the prevalence, and of the deleterious effects of sewer gas, from faulty plumbing, etc.; but they do not insist upon, scarcely indeed mention, the plain fact, that if this insidious destroyer can, as is now known, get into a dwelling through a foot of stone or brick wall, it can and will *get out through an open window*; and that, in any event, if there be abundant ventilation there will be such dilution of these gases as to render them comparatively innoxious. It is not so much the letting in of bad air, but rather the confining of it—the breathing of it, "pure and unadulterated"—that causes disease. There is more *malaria* in a close bedroom in the most favored mountain-region, and in the alimentary canal of a constipated or drug-swallowing dyspeptic, than about the swamps and bayous of Louisiana or the dreaded Roman Campagna, where wrapped in a single blanket, the author has slept night after night—to prove his faith in the theory, as well the theory itself. The "Roman fever," so alarming to visitors of the holy city, is the joint product of stuffy hotel bedrooms and a diet better suited to the climate of Iceland than Italy.

"I have lately spent a summer in a country place whose delicious air is a just source of pride to its inhabitants," says an observing writer, in *Our Continent*. "They told me how doctors sent their patients there from a distance, and how even consumptives had had their fell disease arrested by the tonic effects of the pure air and invigorating breezes, and then I found the very people who thus glorified in them shutting out every breath of air and every ray of sunshine from their houses because of flies! In returning the calls of neighbors, I was struck the moment I entered their houses with that close, unwholesome, 'stuffy' smell which we generally associate with the homes of the ignorant and unneat classes alone, but which is often to be noticed in those of a class far above them. As I looked at the outside of the different houses in the place, it was difficult to realize that they were really inhabited. Every blind was carefully closed, and not one sign of life visible; and yet, unfortunately, life was going on behind those closed windows—life which needed every advantage to make it healthy and enjoyable. Does it never occur to you, you housekeepers whose minds recoil from soiled house-linen, fly-specks on paint, and every species of uncleanliness—does it never occur to you, you so-called neat women, that there is one thing absolutely *dirty* in your cleanly-swept and carefully-dusted houses, and that is their very air? You who would blush with shame at the idea of anything unclean worn on your person, or taken into your mouth, do you not know you are taking in uncleanliness with every breath you draw; and that unclean air is making your blood, and through its means, your entire bodies impure?... Many a woman is regretting this summer that she is unable to have a change of air for herself and children by going to the seaside, the country, or the mountains. Why not try the effect of change of air at home? If air makes such a difference to your health as you admit, why not let it do its best for you wherever you are?"

It would be hard to find, in any community, a person so ignorant as not to know that the lungs require good air. "Oh, yes, of course, I know we must have pure air." Yes, indeed. Nevertheless, ninety-five families in every hundred, in city and country, though always ready to say this, suffer every day of their lives for want of it. This arises from a lack of definite knowledge (1) as to the true office of air—of the fact that it supplies the major portion of the body's nourishment, since an ordinary person could live six weeks or more without eating, and as many days without liquids of any sort; while as many *minutes* without oxygen is certain death; and (2) as to what constitutes "pure air in the home." Says Prof. Huxley: "But the deprivation of oxygen, and the accumulation of carbonic acid, cause injury long before the asphyxiating point is reached. Uneasiness and headache arise when less than one per cent. of the oxygen of the air is replaced by other matters; while the persistent breathing of such air tends to lower all kinds of vital energy, and predisposes to disease. Hence the necessity of sufficient air, and of ventilation for every human being. To be supplied with respiratory air in a *fair state* of purity, every man ought to have at least eight hundred cubic feet of space to himself, and that space ought to be freely accessible, by direct or indirect channels, to the atmosphere."

A room ten feet square, and eight feet high, if "freely accessible" to the outer air during the entire 24 hours, will, according to the high authority quoted, supply the necessary respiratory rations, so to say, for one adult person. In so far, then, as this space *per capita* is diminished, its accessibility to the outer air must be increased; that is, the ventilation (which should in all cases be constant) must be freer, in proportion as the size of the room is diminished or the number of its occupants increased. No room built with hands will ever be large enough to supply the "breath of life," in default of free communication with the outer air.

WINTER VENTILATION.

The true theory of ventilation is to obtain a perpetual and sufficient change of air without sensible draught. The following simple plan, as I have proved by years of experience, perfectly fulfills these requirements, and leaves nothing to be desired. The *Scientific American* endorses the plan, and places it above many, in fact most of the elaborate and expensive devices. The eminent Dr. B. W. Richardson, of London, also, is on record in favor of the plan, and it is already in use in thousands of homes in this country. A three-inch strip placed beneath the lower sash of each window has the effect to "mismatch" the sashes, causing them to overlap each other in the middle.

The stream of air thus admitted is thrown directly upward, and slowly mixes with the heated air in the upper part of the room. As several windows in each room are thus provided, the vitiated air is constantly passing out at one or another of the ventilators. The strip being perfectly fitted or listed, no air can enter at the sill, and all can be so nicely finished as in no manner to mar the appearance of the most elegant drawing-room. A dwelling thus ventilated will never smell "close" to the most sensitive nose upon re-entering, even after a prolonged stay in the open air—a test that would condemn, as unfit for occupancy, ninety in the hundred sitting and sleeping rooms, as well as churches, halls, etc., the world over. The purity of the air is by no means measured by the temperature. Cold air is often very impure by reason of stagnation (as stagnant water), or the exhalations from the lungs, etc., while, on the other hand, the temperature may be maintained at 70° F., or upwards, without fatally lowering its quality, if a sufficient and perpetual change is going on between the outdoor and indoor air.

Whether in Maine or California, Florida or Kansas; whether in a "malarial district" or in a region celebrated for its salubrity,—whatever the locality,—the only standard, the purest air attainable for the inhabitants of any town or hamlet, is the outdoor air. Apropos of this I make a brief extract from the letter of a patient, a delicate lady, under treatment for chronic dyspepsia, and other troubles, who, under date of September 5th, says: "I have tried to follow your directions, and the result is very satisfactory. I live out of doors as much as possible through the day, and for weeks have even slept out on the porch at night. I have enjoyed this very much,—never slept so soundly nor felt so fresh on waking. Of course my friends predicted malaria from sleeping out of doors so near the fogs from the river, but I haven't had even a sniffle! I exercise a great deal and have grown very much stronger. It seemed pretty hard at first to live on one meal a day and exercise too, but I persevered and feel better for it. Every one here is astonished at my progress and increase of strength. At first I think they rather resented my not coming to the table, and they openly declared the foolishness of living without meat; but they have 'sick spells' which now I never do, and they can not endure heat or cold as I can. I think I can dimly see your position, and begin to realize the simplicity of certain problems generally regarded so complicated."—(Mrs. S., Washington, D. C., writing from Wadley's Falls, N. H.)

I feel that my readers will absolve me from the charge of egotism in thus introducing the testimony of this poor lady, the victim of malpractice in the first instance, who, after passing through course after course of drug medication at the hands of eminent, and so-called skillful physicians, at last begins, not dimly, as she herself says, but clearly, as I believe, to see the simplicity of the health question; and especially ought I to be pardoned when I here distinctly remark that I claim to be only the contemporary of thousands upon thousands, physicians and laymen, who have become converts to Hygienic Medicine; being convinced that the proposition is as true as it is simple, that, in general, substances which are injurious for healthy persons to swallow, are even more deleterious to the sick.

CHAPTER XVII.

COFFEE, MEDICINALLY AND DIETETICALLY CONSIDERED.—THE TRUE THEORY OF STIMULATION.[84]

"The chief constituent of the coffee berry, the alkaloid *caffeine*—in chemical analysis recognized as identical with that of the tea plant, *theine*—when separated from the other constituents, ... so as to be seen in its perfect purity, appears in snow-white, silky, filiform crystals, flexible and fragile, without odor, but having a mildly bitter taste.... But it remains an important consideration that this crystallized constituent ... is built on the chemical type of the alkaloid, a class of bodies which nature forms in plants, but not in food-plants—bodies that include narcotics, stimulants, hypnotics, deliriants, poisons, tonics; some of them affecting the whole nervous system, one to excite and another to depress; and others influencing only parts of the nervous system, for special functions of the body."[85]

[84] This paper first appeared in the Boston *Journal of Chemistry* and *Popular Science Review*, May and June, 1882.

[85] Professor Albert B. Prescott, in *Popular Science Monthly*, Jan., 1882, "Chemistry of Tea and Coffee."

"Medically speaking, this theine has a totally distinctive action from the infusions of which it forms a part. In the form of an infusion of tea or coffee, we have to deal with a large proportion of astringent matter, in the form of tannic acid, and with the presence of the essential oil, which is an excitant to the nervous system, and is the substance to which must be ascribed disorders of the nervous system which result from tea and coffee drinking, such as palpitation of the heart and sleeplessness. The theine, upon the other hand, of which there is about one-tenth of a grain in an ordinary cup of tea, is the restorative agent to the nervous system, and is opposed, in its therapeutic properties, to the action of the essential oil. The infusion, therefore, of tea or coffee may induce palpitation in a heart liable to excessive or incoordinate action; but theine, on the contrary, may be looked to, therapeutically, to quiet palpitation. The infusion, by being an excitant, may prevent sleep. Theine, by being a restorative and an indirect sustainer and regulator of the circulation, may induce sleep. Individual medical investigators have, more than this, attempted, from time to time, to show that the action of theine is allied to that of quinine."[86]

[86] "Tea and Coffee as Nervines," by Dr. Lewis Shapter, in *British Medical Journal*.

It can not be questioned that the administration of coffee, in the form of an infusion or otherwise, is entirely in accord with the theory and practice of medicine at the present day. It is, however, a fact well known to practitioners, and indeed generally to "laymen," that the constant and long-continued use of any medicine transforms its "remedial" influence into one promotive of disease that may perhaps demand the curative aid of some other drug.

A strong infusion of *café noir* (administered, it is to be presumed, to one not an habitual user) has been recently claimed by a celebrated French physician as an effectual antidote for the blood-poison that exists in typhus, typhoid, and yellow fevers. While this may be true, I am sure that there are, on the other hand, good grounds for the belief that the habitual use of coffee as an article of diet aids materially in the accumulation of the poison, and in the production of that abnormal condition or quality of the tissues of the body which the vital forces seek to rectify by means of the expulsive efforts which constitute the symptoms of typhoid and other fevers. Indeed, Dr. Segur, who evidently regards coffee as the nearest approach to the Elixir of Life, claims, as one of the *benefits* resulting from its use, that "it lessens the waste of tissue, and therefore renders less food necessary." Now, to interfere with or hinder any of the normal processes of the organism, especially those most vital to the economy, as, for example, that of the constant breaking down and excretion of the tissues, is not only to invite, but the impairment of these functions in and of itself constitutes, disease. He further says, "After a heavy meal, it relieves the sense of oppression and helps digestion." What it really accomplishes, however, in such cases, is this: it mitigates the immediate effects of excess by diluting and washing away a portion of the food (of course unprepared for intestinal digestion), and, after the first congestive effects have subsided, by producing anæmia of the stomach, thereby *hindering* digestion, it relieves temporarily, but at great cost ultimately, the sense of oppression produced by a gluttonous meal. By hindering digestion, in this or in any other manner, as, for example, by resuming muscular or mental labor directly after eating, we may prevent or delay plethora—the surcharge of the blood with nutritive material that results from the rapid absorption of an over-full meal;[87] but later on there will take place in the alimentary tract more or less fermentation of its undigested contents, which, with the foul and noxious gases generated thereby, will, to a greater or less degree, be absorbed into the circulation. Thus we observe the two-fold effect of this most delicious and seductive beverage: by "lessening the waste," it prevents the body from remaining sound in its tissues, (see index: "fossil bodies") and causes blood-poisoning from indigestion. For if, by reason of anæmia of the stomach and intestines, the digestive fluids are not secreted in sufficient amount to preserve it, "the food rapidly undergoes chemical decomposition in the alimentary canal, and often putrefies."[88] This accounts for the gas coming from the stomach and bowels of persons troubled with indigestion and constipation, who frequently complain of a rotten-egg taste in the mouth. "This gas, in its poisonous effect, is similar to hydrocyanic or prussic acid, only not so powerful. It is a very destructive agent in its interference with those vital processes concerned in ultimate nutrition, robbing the blood corpuscles of vitality, and preventing the transformation into tissue of the nutriment conveyed by the circulation, and of worn-out tissue into waste, thus poisoning the blood and nervous centers, and disturbing the whole animal economy." In view of this state of things, need we search with microscopes for the causes of sickness, go outside of our own bodies for "malaria," or look to any extraordinary circumstance as essential to generate the most deadly diseases? According to the recent experiments (on dogs) of M. Lennen, communicated to the Paris Society of Biology, coffee does produce "anæmia of the stomach, retards digestion, and, the anæmia repeating itself, ends by bringing on habitual increased congestion of the stomach, which, according to M. Lennen, is synonymous with dyspepsia."

[87] As explained elsewhere (p. 201), gentle exercise in the open air, after such a meal, though not the best, is nevertheless a remedy.

[88] Effects of Excess in Diet, "Physiology and Hygiene," p. 402, Huxley.

It is not difficult, then, to comprehend why the final effect of coffee must be especially injurious, if not disastrous, to asthmatics and "consumptives," the head and front of whose disease is dyspepsia, pure and simple. (See "Consumption.") The *British Medical Journal*, after noting the experiments of M. Lennen, and favoring his conclusions, goes on to say: "It is well known—and English physicians have laid great stress upon this point—that the abuse of coffee and tea often brings on gastralgia, dyspepsia, and, at the same time, more or less disturbance of the *apparatus of innervation*." The question naturally arises, What constitutes an "abuse" of a medicine? I should say its daily use as a beverage.

Coffee is a *purgative*—a very agreeable form of breakfast pill—but, as with all purgative medicines, an increasing dose is necessary, and its final effect is constipation, with no end of possibilities as a result of the retention of waste matters in the blood. Constipation, however produced, is a *predisposing* cause, and the continuance of the habits that have produced and now maintain it constitutes a sufficient *exciting* cause, of such diseases as neuralgia, rheumatism, erysipelas, fevers of various sorts (including scarlet fever and "head cold,") and, with the aid of sewer gas *insufficiently diluted with outdoor air*—by means of ventilation—diphtheria, or any of the zymotic "diseases." Worst of all, those more terrible maladies (because more permanent and enduring, and unrecognized as symptoms of disease), as nervousness, peevishness, irritability, and general unreasonableness, are due, in great measure, to impoverishment of the blood; the nerves are insufficiently nourished, and the brain is "set on edge" by the poisoned circulation.

Professor Prescott makes this very interesting remark with regard to the chemistry of coffee and tea: "But the change of guanine into theine is easily accomplished. It is perfectly practicable to bring guano material to the laboratory, and send away the same atomic elements transformed into the snow-white, silky crystals of theine. Given only sufficient demand for the pure stimulant principle of tea and coffee, and a market high enough above the cost of its vegetable sources, and it might then safely be predicted that not many months would elapse before companies with thousands of capital stock would engage successfully in the chemical manufacture of theine from guano. Then, very likely, rival companies would establish the claim to manufacture a still purer article from certain of the waste substances of the world—articles more accessible than guano."

As to the nutritive properties of coffee, although the food constituents of the *berry* are considerable in quantity, yet so deficient are they in digestibility that, in the infusion especially, it is more than doubtful if they are of advantage in supporting life, under any circumstances; indeed, I have no doubt that the poisonous effects of the alkaloid and tannin far outweigh any gain from the nutrients. At any rate, he would be a bold man, indeed, and I doubt not a defeated one in the end, who should attempt to imitate Mr. John Griscomb's fast of forty-five days (which was attended by no discomfort even), substituting coffee infusion for pure water.

Coffee interferes with digestion, and, consequently, with nutrition, aside from its specific or general effects upon the digestive organs, by the manner in which it is usually taken: a mouthful of food and then a draught of the beverage prevents the necessity of chewing[89] and prohibits the secretion of the saliva and its admixture with the starchy elements of the cereals and vegetables, so essential to the preparation of this class of food for digestion further on. The first process in the transformation of starch into blood, is its conversion into grape sugar, and we know that saliva fulfills this function; and while it is believed that the intestinal juices also act in the same manner, still, we are not at liberty to suppose that the preliminary change designed to be begun in the mouth is unnecessary. Or, if it be in a measure true that this fluid, being constantly secreted and swallowed, *thus* performs its legitimate function, it is certain that the salivary glands are injured, their functions impaired, and the quality and quantity of their secretions modified by the ingestion of hot, astringent fluids; and this must certainly be one of the injurious effects of tobacco-chewing or smoking. No one would suppose for one moment that the glands of the liver, or kidneys, for example, could continue their offices satisfactorily in face of constant contact with a poultice of tobacco, corresponding in size to an ordinary quid, which would, in the mouth of a novice, produce purgative effects, often within one minute from its application. In fact, it may be relied upon that the ingestion into the mouth or stomach of any substance that causes the bowels to "act," in the common understanding of this term, whether the dose be in solid or liquid form—tends to, and the constant or frequent use of such devices will, impair and permanently injure the entire alimentary tract, from mouth to anus, and all its secreting and excreting glands.

[89] The prevalence of "bad teeth" is in my opinion referable chiefly to three causes: (1) innutrition resulting from the use of impoverished or indigestible food substance, (2) the use of hot drinks, (3) *non-use* of the teeth; dental exercise is the best dentifrice. Observe the quality, whiteness and clean condition of the dogs' teeth: from early youth their "tooth-brushes" are bones, which they are constantly gnawing. Bread-crusts, or wheat-kernels, would do the business for our young growing children, replacing "candy," for instance.

Coffee is a *diuretic*, and hence its habitual use promotes disease of the kidneys. "Very warm drinks are in themselves debilitating to the stomach, but the addition of the properties of tea, coffee, or other herbs, burdens the kidneys and urinary apparatus with an unnatural amount of labor continually. (See Bright's Disease.) These organs, kept constantly over-excited, must become debilitated, and preternaturally irritable, and this condition of debility and irritability extends sympathetically to all the surrounding viscera; finally, the abdominal muscles themselves become relaxed, and, with the general nervous exhaustion produced by the active nervine and narcotic properties of the herb throughout the system, a foundation is laid for the whole train of maladies, displacements of organs, disordered functions, and 'weaknesses,' which are so general at the present day."

Again, coffee is often referred to as a respiratory food. It does, in small doses, and at first, have the effect to excite abnormally the nerves governing the respiratory movements, as well as those of the heart, stomach, etc.—stimulates them; hence the tendency, finally, to sluggish action of these organs, and even paralysis: a peculiar type of "nightmare" often met with among coffee and tobacco users, illustrates this well, although the connection is not usually comprehended,—a feeling of suffocation, following one of pressure, or "rushing feeling," at the base of the brain, as it is often described; usually observed at night just as the individual is dropping off to sleep, seemingly at the very moment of "losing" himself, and very naturally, too, at this particular moment: prior thereto there had been somewhat of a constrained feeling, perhaps, unobserved by the victim, who, while awake, would continue the process of breathing by means of an unconscious, but still real, degree of voluntary effort. In sleep, the suffocation which ensues causes the victim to wake with a start and with a violent palpitation of the heart; or he may not succeed in rousing himself: this means death. In fact, all stimulants and poisons, as tobacco, coffee, distilled liquors, etc., *tend* to local and general paralysis.

Coffee is styled the drink, *par excellence*, of the brain-worker. Cases like the following are by no means rare: Under the influence of two or three cups of strong coffee the brain of an essayist works satisfactorily, perhaps for hours; the hands and feet meanwhile growing cold and clammy, and the entire surface "chilly," while the brain throbs with congestion, until, finally, the mind becomes confused, strange mistakes are made, words are repeated or misspelled, and although the over-stimulated but now clogged and exhausted brain can see, dimly outlined within itself, pages, whole chapters perhaps, that must be written now or be forever lost—or at least his diseased imagination thus pictures it—still he finds it impossible to proceed, and with a martyr spirit, or perhaps despairingly, he ceases from his labors. A night of disturbed sleep (see article on Insomnia) almost surely follows, and during its waking intervals the brain often does its best work, which is worse than lost, unless the sufferer rises in (what should be) "the dead hours of the night" to record his brilliant thoughts. This effort he is often loath to make: he can think, or rather can not stop thinking, but he feels too weak to rise. Imperfect, however, as may be his repose, still, he may, with the aid of fresh stimulation, be enabled to take up his work again for the day. This may go on indefinitely, but with less and less satisfactory results from month to month,—neuralgic pains, "nervous headaches," or other evidence of visceral irritation, meantime adding to the sufferings to be endured,—until, after a time, becoming alarmed, he feels the need of a long vacation. If, however, in spite of all premonitions of danger, he keeps on denying himself the "rest" (from stimulation as well as from labor) he so much needs, it is like pulling a heavy load up-hill, and a little later he finds himself utterly prostrated. Whether, now, he dies speedily of paralysis, "heart disease," or "nervous prostration"; fails gradually and dies of "consumption"; or recovers some degree of health, after a long illness, the cause of his disease is believed by himself, friends—and physician, perhaps—to have been "overwork."[90] In fact, it is the effect of *stimulation* inciting to excessive brain, to the neglect of physical, exercise; the brain is clogged by its own unexcreted waste, and the entire system unbalanced and unstrung. It is in such cases that a resort to "tonic treatment," beef-tea, or a "generous diet" of flesh-food—for which, perhaps, a fictitious appetite is created by the use of "regular" or irregular bitters—often destroys the patient's last chance for recovery. "It is," says Professor Brunton, "piling on fuel, instead of removing ash."[91]

[90] The same amount of the stimulant alone (coffee, tobacco, wine, or what not), *without* the hard work that tended to aid in its elimination, would have made quicker work of it. What such a person requires under these circumstances is to give his brain rest from severe mental application. Nor is it, in my opinion, sound doctrine to say that a weary-brained man may rest by rushing at muscular exercise, or *vice versa*. To a certain extent the rule holds good; but the exhausted or very tired man requires a period of absolute rest, before taking up any form of work. At the proper time, however, he will be improved by taking up active exercise in the open air, and performing daily such regular muscular and literary work as he can comfortably, however little this may be, without any sort of stimulation other than that derived from simple, nutritious food and pure air. (See article on Consumption for hint as to exercise.)

[91] "Indigestion as a Cause of Nervous Prostration," *Popular Science Monthly*, January, 1881.

The illustration here given is one of the worst cases, but such instances are frequently observed among the class usually designated as brain workers, not only, but among business men, whose work, scheming, mishaps, and unnatural habits altogether, bring them to sick-beds and premature graves; while mild forms are met with constantly everywhere.

Whatever degree of eminence our brain-workers may hope to attain under any form of stimulation, before their lives shall be prematurely ended, all may rest assured that by obeying the laws of life and building up a healthy body they will, in the long run—the "run" made longer thereby—do more and better work without than with artificial aid. The stimulus of good health is far better than that derived from any stimulating drink. The most brilliant productions of the brain, under stimulation, may, strictly speaking, be called *premature births*.

Professor Proctor, in the paper before alluded to, further says: "Notwithstanding the adoption of theine-containing beverages by mankind at large, we can not hesitate to commend that robust habit which discards all dependence on adventitious food, even on so mild a stimulus as that of the tea-cup, and preserves through life the fresh integrity of full nervous susceptibility. And probably there was never a time when there were so many persons as now who are disposed, by conviction and by a desire for a stalwart physical independence, to refuse to fix any habit that holds the nervous system."

Dr. Segur asserts that "habitual coffee-drinkers generally enjoy good health and live to a good old age." We find, however, that a very large proportion of those coffee-drinkers who are observing and conscientious freely confess to the ill effects of the beverage: It makes them "nervous, irritable, or gives them headache frequently," they say; and it is quite common to hear them declare that they would leave it off if they could, but they "depend on it—it is the principal part of breakfast." Often enough it is all the breakfast taken. It prevents hunger or appeases it by rendering the stomach anæmic, and its stimulating effects are mistaken for added strength. And it is even worse where the coffee-drinker is at the same time a full-feeder; for, are we not told that this beverage "lessens the waste of tissue and renders less food necessary?" Quite a percentage of even robust people, beginning to feel, or to recognize after having long felt, the twinges of dyspepsia do, either on their own judgment or by the advice of the family physician, give up the habit, and find great benefit from the change; and but for clinging to other unnatural practices, they might often bid adieu to all their physical ills.

A few, comparatively, of the most vigorous men and women, it can not be denied, do "enjoy good health and live to a good old age," in spite of many injurious practices, including the habitual use of the stimulant coffee. But even these have their intervals of suffering, more or less severe —"attacks" that better habits would prevent. Of the latter class, out of scores whom I might mention, the experience of O. B. Frothingham is noteworthy. He says: "Although no positive ill effect has been traceable to either of them [tea and coffee] or wine, all of which have been used sparingly, yet, were my life to live over again, I should accustom myself to abstinence from all three. It seems to me now, on looking back, that something of dullness and languor, something of exhaustion and dreaminess, something of lethargy, something too of heat and irritability, may be chargeable to a practice not in any grave degree harmful or blameworthy. The faculties have been less keen and patient than they would have been under a strictly natural regimen."

It might, perhaps, in this connection, be profitable to ask,

WHAT IS A "STIMULANT"?

In reply I would say that any poisonous or unnatural substance ingested into the living body, in amount within the ability of the vital organism to *readily* expel it; or even of the most wholesome food substance in excess of the *needs* of the organism, and yet, again, not so excessive as to depress the vital forces instead of spurring them to increased efforts to thrust it out, is a stimulant. In short, anything of an injurious nature, by reason of quality, amount, or the conditions under which it is administered, may produce stimulating effects. But the inevitable "reaction" of stimulation is depression; although, from natural causes, convalescents often make sufficient progress to overwhelm, or at least obscure, the evidence of the secondary effects.

Speaking with direct reference to the effect of alkaloids in general, Professor Prescott says, "While a certain portion stimulates the nervous system, a large portion acts as a sedative, so that a difference in quantity of the potion causes a difference in kind of its effects." It should ever be borne in mind that the increased action under stimulation is simply the extra effort forced upon the vital organism to expel an intruder—the intruder being the stimulant itself. If this be the case, it necessarily follows that stimulants deplete, and can never replenish the vital exchequer. Instances have been noted of children who were observed to be unusually active and jubilant immediately prior to an "attack" of diphtheria. In such case—and a true history of every case might establish this as the rule—the diphtheritic poison acts as a stimulant; nature is trying to thrust it out, and all the life forces are abnormally active. We can not know in how many instances she succeeds in these efforts, nor yet how often her defeats are due to the administration of poisons, and food that for want of digestion becomes a poison, altogether so adding to the toxic condition that nature finally ends an evil she can not cure. After a vigorous expulsive efforts, for example, the system, temporarily quiescent, gathering fresh strength for a renewal of the conflict to dislodge the enemy, or, possibly, having already accomplished the main work, now rests in the stage preceding convalescence—is supposed to require the aid of a stimulant, and food also must be given at frequent intervals "to prevent the patient from sinking;" but alas, this proves the weight about his neck that carries him to the bottom—"supported" to death. In comparing the stimulation of the vital organism, in sickness, to the spurring up of a tired or lazy animal to greater exertion, there is always this grand difference: the former will every time, and always, exert its entire force, that is, will exert it better, more savingly to life, without, than with, stimulation. "Self-preservation is the first law of nature;" and no other circumstance possible to imagine, better illustrates this law, than the living organism in sickness.

Coffee makes the timid or diffident man brave—gives him confidence in himself; but, by "reaction," this fictitious bravery gives place to nervousness. Many persons experience a certain undefinable dread of approaching danger, a veritable "can't-sleep-for-fear-of-burglars" sort of wakefulness, which leaves them after a few weeks' abstinence from coffee-stimulation. Hot coffee or tea makes one warm—the very finger-tips tingle with warm blood; but later, in default of another dram—perhaps in spite of it—he feels chilly, even in a warm room; there is a "can't-get-warm-any-way" sort of feeling, to be accounted for, he fancies, only upon the theory that he has "caught cold!" He is suffering from coffee poisoning.

Although personally a dear lover of coffee, and, by reason of an exceptionally robust habit of body, at present, able to indulge in its use with less apparent harm than I find, upon long and careful inquiry and observation, is the case with most people, yet, nevertheless, I stand condemned by the eulogy of Abd-el-Kadir Anasari Dgezeri Hambali, son of Mahomet: "O coffee! thou dispellest the cares of the great; thou bringest back those who wander from the paths of knowledge. Coffee is the beverage of the people of God, and the cordial of his servants who thirst for wisdom. When coffee is infused into the bowl, it exhales the *odor of musk*, and is of the *color of ink*. The truth is not known except to the wise, who drink it from the foaming coffee-cup. God has deprived fools of coffee, who, with invincible obstinacy, condemn it as injurious."

According to Professor Prescott, "the administration of theine in small portions, to animals or to man, quickens the circulation and effects some degree of mental exhilaration and wakefulness. In final result, the excretion of carbonic-acid gas is diminished, and the flow of blood through the capillaries is retarded." "Larger portions," he continues, "prove poisonous, causing painful restlessness, rigidity of the muscles, and general exhaustion. Not more than three or four grains at once can be properly taken for medicinal or experimental purposes." As often prepared for old coffee-tipplers, two cupfuls (about 16 oz.) of the infusion will contain this quantity of the alkaloid. As usually taken, of course, the proportion of the alkaloid is much less. In conclusion, I would repeat that it may with propriety be claimed for coffee that its administration as a medicine is as legitimate as that of any other, and no more so; certainly its daily use as an article of diet is as inconsistent and contrary to reason, as the similar use of any drug in the materia medica.

Note.—In the foregoing I have not considered the question of the influence of tea and coffee upon the "temperance movement." One of the keenest observers of human nature, as well as one of our soundest *thinkers*, Dr. Oswald, from whose Physical Education I have freely drawn in the chapters on Consumption—and his view in this matter is endorsed by many very able physiologists and sociologists—says (p. 64): "The road to the rum-cellar leads through the coffee-house. Abstinence from *all* stimulants, only, is easier than temperance." Everywhere do I find temperance reformers essaying to lead rum-drinkers back *by the road they came,* viz: back through the coffee-house—taking a drink *en route*. I think that, in the long run, they will do better to try to conduct them from the "gin-mill" squarely into the street, and thence home. While not desiring to furnish arguments for the opponents of temperance (I would that *all* stimulants were done away with), I cannot forbear pointing out what seems to me a glaring inconsistency among my co-laborers in reform. Of course all must admit that, in many respects, there can be no comparison drawn between liquor-drinking and tea and coffee-drinking: Other things equal, the man who drinks "rum" to excess, works vastly more misery in the world than the coffee toper; though, individually, if the latter were to indulge as copiously as does his spirit-drinking contemporary, he would suffer as much, probably more, in his health—would die more speedily. Of course we know that few coffee and tea-drinkers indulge to this extreme; but when we consider the almost universal use of these beverages—by women and growing children, as well as by men, it is more than doubtful whether they do not, *per se*, from a health point of view (considering, moreover, the influence of disease upon morals) aggregate more harm than their *more* "ardent" rivals. Added to this, the fact that the use of one stimulant often leads to the use of others and stronger (as we have always argued that beer and wine lead on to whisky and brandy), the friends of true reform may well ask themselves whether, in their own indulgence in tea and coffee, and in the effort to increase their use among the people, they are not hitting wide of the mark? I am well aware that wine-drinkers, and those who indulge moderately in stronger drink, often pertinently reply to temperance workers, "When all the temperance reformers leave off *their* favorite stimulants we will leave off ours." Says Dr. Dudley A. Sargent, Professor of Physical Culture at Harvard College, "I am convinced that coffee works more injury to mankind than beer."

CHAPTER XVIII.

APPETITE—CONTINENCE.

Appetite, in a general sense, means a natural degree of hunger (not craving), sufficient to give relish for any kind of wholesome food. "We often hear people say they have no taste for this or that article of plain food, although many such have an insatiable appetite for all the dainties of the table. Morbid appetites are thus engendered by continuous habits of indulgence. Natural appetites are first enfeebled and then vitiated; health of body is slowly and insidiously impaired, until, by and by, innate nobility and hopeful youth and strength become effeminate, fastidious, weak, irascible, and selfish; and though outwardly, perhaps, refined and delicate, the person inwardly becomes inactive, apathetic, and unhelpful to himself and to the world. The natural sun of heat and life within the body and the soul, being overcast by the clouds and exhalations of unhealthy organs, often leads the victim of self-indulgence to seek externally for artificial stimulants to keep up an appearance of genial warmth within—but this can only be apparently successful for a time; and soon the penalty of the transgression of the laws of nature must be paid in full, and with, a large additional amount of costs. It is of great importance, therefore, to watch the appetites of body and of mind; to study the laws of healthy equilibrium; and, above all, to learn to know and understand the dangers of prolonged self-indulgence of the appetites of pleasure in mere animal sensation and wild imagination. Appetite, properly so called, apprises man of the natural wants of the organism, and compliance with these internal promptings is rewarded by the double pleasure of the sense of taste in eating, and the feeling of comfort within, arising from the food supplied to the digestive system. But where the mind is weak and the delights of bodily sensation strong, the pleasures of taste or the charm of varied sensations in the palate dwell on the imagination and excite it to renewed indulgence of physical sensations, irrespective of the wants of the internal organism, and this even notwithstanding its declining health and manifest debility." The morbid cravings of the sense of perverted taste, or any other sense, must not be confounded, therefore, with the natural appetite excited by the wants of the internal organism. "In the bear tribes there is a marked preference for honey manifested, which reveals a sense of taste that works on the imagination, and leads him to incur the risk of being stung to death by an infuriated swarm of bees rather than forego the sensual delights of plundering the hive and licking out the honeycomb when he is master of the spoils. The swollen head and face and ears are nothing to the charm of sensual indulgence." When I observe the sufferers from sick-headache or neuralgia (see Rheumatism), with swollen face and bandaged head, I am forcibly reminded of the honey-loving bear.

No expert can observe the habits of the people and fail to account for all the diseases that afflict the human family. Victims of disobedience to the natural laws—they have done the things they ought not to have done, and have left undone the things they ought to have done, and (consequently) there is no health in them. Diseases—how slowly we accept their teaching—how blind we are to their warning voice! The word itself is not understood. The term disease is popularly applied only to the most serious forms, such as have been named, when it is properly applicable to any condition other than the normal condition of the body—perfect ease. Acidity, heartburn, flatulence, slight pains in the head, uneasy sensations of whatever sort—so little regarded until too late—are they not dis-ease? They speak plainly of indigestion,—the causes of which are recited elsewhere;—they are to the body what the degree-points are to the thermometer, and require only to be conscientiously considered to ensure freedom from disturbance.

Other appetites there are which become morbid and too often control the individual, instead of being themselves under entire subjection to him.

The unnatural habits of our civilization have caused the race to depart from the natural instinct of

CONTINENCE

which, to the minds of many, is as essential to the moral and physical health of the race after, as to its "virtue" before, marriage; and which, but for the inflammatory nature of the diet in general use, and the disorders arising therefrom, might easily be practiced by all conscientious and thoughtful people. A radical modification of the prevailing dietetic practices would lessen, immeasurably, the constant warfare between the moral desires and the animal propensities, to which both the married and the single are subjected, and which results in disaster in so many instances. "Marital excesses often produce in the offspring sexual precocity and passions which, under the influence of an unwholesome and stimulating dietary, are rendered ungovernable, and entail a vast deal of shame and sorrow throughout the lives of those who are 'more sinned against than sinning.' Verily the sins of the parents shall be visited upon the children even to the third and fourth generation of them that hate Him and violate His law."[92]

[92] Chapter on "Health Hints" in "How To Feed The Baby."

"Ah! my friends," said the Rev. F. W. Farrar, Canon of Westminster Abbey, "how vast a part of human disease results, not only from the ignorance but also from the folly and sin of man. Typhoid, leprosy, small-pox, and jail-fever are not by any means the only diseases which might be almost, if not quite, eliminated from among us. We talk with deep self-pity of the ravages of gout and cancer and consumption and mental alienation. *Alas! how many of these might in one or two generations cease to be, if we all lived the wise and temperate and happy lives which Nature meant us to lead!* And the voice of Nature, rightly interpreted, is ever the voice of God. Even the simplest of us are superfluous in our demands, and the vast majority of men so live as, more or less, habitually to pamper the appetite by wasteful extravagance and weaken the health by baneful luxuries. By unwholesome narcotics, by burning and adulterated stimulants, by many and highly-seasoned meats, by thus storing the blood with unnatural elements which it can not assimilate, they clog and carnalize the aspirations which they should cherish, and feed into uncontrollable force the passions which they should control. Hence it is that millions of lives are like sweet bells jangled out of tune; and millions of men in these days, like the Israelites of old, are laid to rest in *Kibroth Hattaavah*—the graves of lust!

"And the sad thing is that this heavy punishment ends not with the individual. It is not only that the boy when he has marred his own boyhood, hands on its moral results to the youth; and the youth when he has marred them yet more irretrievably hands them on to the man that he may finish the task of that perdition;—but alas! the man also hands them on to his innocent children, and they are born with bodies tormented with the disproportionate impulses, sickly with the morbid cravings, enfeebled by the increasing degeneracy, tainted by the retributive disease of guilty parents."

We must remember, says Albert Leffingwell, quoting the above in "Laws of Life," that he who speaks thus is no obscure Boanerges, vaguely ranting over abstract sin, but one of the few great preachers in the Church of England, speaking in the most venerable religious edifice in Protestant Christendom.

The most persistent and thorough cramming of our youth with high moral precepts avails but little, after all,—we observe this constantly,—to counteract the fierce impulses of an unbalanced physical state.

Says the Duke of Argyle: "The truth is, that we are born into a system of things in which every act carries with it, by indissoluble ties, a long train of consequences reaching to the most distant future, and which for the whole course of time affect our own condition, the condition of other men, and even the conditions of external nature. And yet we can not see those consequences beyond the shortest way, and very often those which lie nearest are in the highest degree deceptive as an index to ultimate results.

Neither pain nor pleasure can be accepted as a guide. With the lower animals, indeed, these, for the most part tell the truth, the whole truth, and nothing but the truth. Appetite is all that the creature has, and in the gratification of it the highest law of the animal being is fulfilled. In man, too, appetite has its own indispensable function to discharge. But it is a lower function, and amounts to nothing more than that of furnishing to Reason a few of the primary data on which it has to work—a few, and a few only. Physical pain is indeed one of the threatenings of natural authority; and physical pleasure is one of its rewards. But neither the one nor the other forms more than a mere fraction of that awful and imperial code under which we live. It is the code of an everlasting kingdom, and of a jurisprudence which endures throughout all ages." ... "It is no mere failure to realize aspirations which are vague and imaginary that constitutes this exceptional element (the persistent tendency of his development to take a wrong direction) in the history and in the actual conditions of mankind. That which constitutes the terrible anomaly of his case admits of perfectly clear and specific definition. Man has been and still is a constant prey to appetites which are morbid—to opinions which are irrational, to imaginings which are horrible, and to practices which are destructive. The prevalence and the power of these in a great variety of forms and of degrees is a fact with which we are familiar—so familiar, indeed, that we fail to be duly impressed with the strangeness and the mystery which really belong to it. All savage races are bowed and bent under the yoke of their own perverted instincts—instincts which generally in their root and origin have an obvious utility, but which in their actual development are the source of miseries without number and without end. Some of the most horrible perversions which are prevalent among savages, (and which to a greater or less degree affect all civilized peoples), have no counterpart among any other created beings, and when judged by the barest standard of utility, place man immeasurably below the level of the beasts. We are accustomed to say of many of the habits of savage life that they are 'brutal.' But this is entirely to misrepresent the place which they really occupy in the system of Nature. None of the brutes have any such perverted dispositions; none of them are ever subject to the destructive operation of such habits as are common among men. And the contrast is all the more remarkable when we consider that the very worst of these habits affect conditions of life which the lower animals share with us, and in which any departure from those natural laws which they universally obey, must necessarily produce, and do actually produce, consequences so destructive as to endanger the very existence of the race. Such are all those conditions of life affecting the relation of the sexes which are common to all creatures, and in which man alone exhibits the widest and most hopeless divergence from the order of Nature."

CHAPTER XIX.

CONCLUSION.

While the more important material agencies and conditions, closely related to the processes of life, are air, food, clothing, etc.; and while the reader's attention has been, throughout, mainly directed to these; it would, from the author's point of view, constitute a serious defect of the work, to omit the special consideration of the moral nature—its mighty influence over the physical state. In no better way can I impress this thought than by quoting the language of that veteran hygienist and reformer, Dr. James C. Jackson:

"But while a human being has a physical organization, and has, therefore, physical laws, he is dual, possessing also a spiritual nature; and to treat him for any disease he may have as though it originated in his body and did not relate itself at all to his soul or spirit, is to treat him, in ninety-nine cases in a hundred, unphilosophically and therefore unscientifically. Our observation and experience go to satisfy us that the majority of sick persons become disturbed and disordered in spirit before they show disorder or derangement of body.

"To illustrate: a man never comes to be a dyspeptic until he has a false spiritual conception of the true relations which he should hold to the use of food; he is conceptively sick before he is physically dyspeptic; he turns things right around in his mind; he lives to eat instead of eating to live; he is spiritually depraved before he becomes physically diseased. Take the methods of life common to our people. It is largely through these that they become sick. They eat badly, drink badly, dress unhealthfully, work without reference to their power to recover from the fatigue which work imposes, do not get sleep enough, are in a fret, or in a worry, or in a strife, or are under strain in their work. They work selfishly or for their own good only, and often as against the good of others; they seek to thrive at others' unthrift; they buy and sell with the view in their minds of living gainfully at others' loss; they have a false conception, a perverse view, of the relationships which they should hold to others, and under this spiritual perversity they put forth their energies. As they are inwardly wrong they become outwardly disordered, and when this disorder develops into actual sickness it has a spiritual or wrong moral basis. Having violated the higher law of their natures, in selfishness of thought and feeling, they are compelled to take the reflex effects in and upon their bodies. Living without sympathy, they become sympathetically diseased; the sympathetic forces in their nature, lacking proper expression or use, become debilitated and deranged, as shown in the abnormal condition of the sympathetic nervous structure.

"For instance: a man with his liver functionally deranged appears before a physician: The pulse shows the circulation to be disturbed; the excretory system has become largely inactive—the skin, bowels, kidneys, and lungs each working inefficiently or compelled to overdo. The doctor concludes that a good dose of calomel and jalap, which enter into the allopathic practice; or some sitz-baths, skin-rubbing, packs, or injections, which would be the hydropathic practice; or regulation of diet, connected with some mild alterative, which belong to the eclectic practice; or some little pills, which would be the homœopathic practice, are what the man needs. He is a glutton, or a wine-bibber, or he drinks whiskey, or he lives bodily not only, but morally and spiritually on the line of self-indulgence. He lives as he pleases, and this not merely in his animal life. He lives spiritually as he pleases; his spirit is selfish and lawless. Order and righteousness are not in all his thoughts. His conscience is asleep; his intelligence is not at all on the alert; he has no inspirations, or aspirations; he simply has unhallowed desires, and his life consists largely in efforts to gratify these, and there he is—disturbed, disordered, deranged, diseased, sick.

"When one thus affected comes to us, what do we do with him? We bring him to judgment; we summon him up into the presence of the truth. We say: You are at fault for this sickness of yours; it is not necessary for you to be sick; you may be a healthy person, you should be. You may be free from aches and pains, you ought to be. There is no defectiveness in your organization; it is made to run successfully; that it does not, is your fault, not the fault of your circumstances. What you need is right perception and a good conscience to back it; a willingness, not only, but a thorough will to do right. In you is ample vital force to set your liver right, make your bowels work, make your skin carry on its insensible perspiration, your blood circulate healthfully, and have everything done according to law. All that is necessary is that you put your spirit, your responsible consciousness on the throne, and make your body its servant. When you resolve to do this and begin to do it, you will begin to get well. You do not need medicine; you need nothing done for you in order to get well, except to do judiciously, and, in your conditions, discretely, what if you had done all the while would have kept you well.

"The first thing to do is, not to consult doctors: not to hunt for some wonderful curative; but to get right ideas of life, and then begin, though in a feeble manner, to conform yourself to that way spiritually. *Love* the thing you are going to do; get your whole nature into a glow toward it. If it be to eat simple food, love to do it—not do it wishing you had not to do it. Look at the thing kindly, joyfully, comfortingly. Put away your evil habits, one after another, because they are evil, not simply because they hurt you. Get up a rebellion in your spirit against wrong ways of living. Resolve that you will not live wrongly; characterize that way as it should be characterized, as an improper, unmanly, mean, or unbefitting way for you. Say: I will not smoke; I will not drink; I will not make my body an instrument of gluttony; and so go through your whole round of habits, putting away all those that you can get along without. Reduce your artificial wants to a minimum.

Throw yourself over on the line of order and law, and regularity and propriety. Then you will get well."

www.ingramcontent.com/pod-product-compliance
Lightning Source LLC
Chambersburg PA
CBHW081156020426
42333CB00020B/2527